The Joint Commission

Toolkit for New Accreditation Professionals

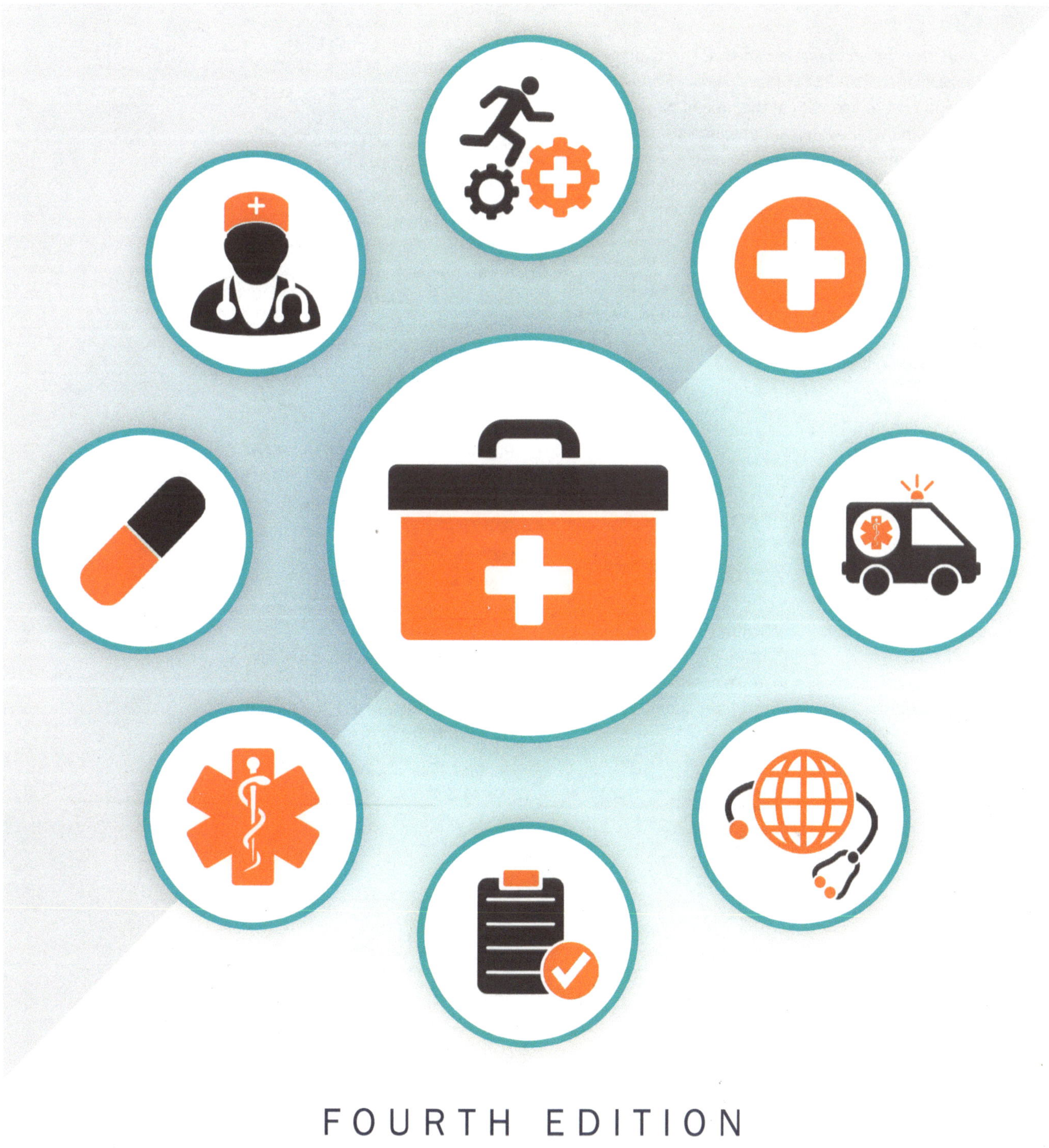

FOURTH EDITION

JOINT COMMISSION RESOURCES MISSION

The mission of Joint Commission Resources (JCR) is to continuously improve the safety and quality of health care in the United States and in the international community through the provision of education, publications, consultation, and evaluation services.

DISCLAIMERS

JCR educational programs and publications support, but are separate from, the accreditation activities of The Joint Commission. Attendees at Joint Commission Resources educational programs and purchasers of JCR publications receive no special consideration or treatment in, or confidential information about, the accreditation process. The inclusion of an organization name, product, or service in a JCR publication should not be construed as an endorsement of such organization, product, or service, nor is failure to include an organization name, product, or service to be construed as disapproval.

This publication is designed to provide accurate and authoritative information regarding the subject matter covered. Every attempt has been made to ensure accuracy at the time of publication; however, please note that laws, regulations, and standards are subject to change. Please also note that some of the examples in this publication are specific to the laws and regulations of the locality of the facility. The information and examples in this publication are provided with the understanding that the publisher is not engaged in providing medical, legal, or other professional advice. If any such assistance is desired, the services of a competent professional person should be sought.

Joint Commission Resources
Oakbrook Terrace, Illinois 60181
https://www.jcrinc.com

Joint Commission Resources, Inc. (JCR), a not-for-profit affiliate of The Joint Commission, has been designated by The Joint Commission to publish publications and multimedia products. JCR reproduces and distributes these materials under license from The Joint Commission.

ISBN (print): 978-1-63585-384-1
ISBN (e-book): 978-1-63585-385-8

Printed in the USA

For more information about The Joint Commission, please visit **https://www.jointcommission.org**.

DEVELOPMENT TEAM

Senior Editor: Margaret McConnell
Associate Director, Accreditation Content: Mary Beth Curran
Associate Director, Editorial, Books/Digital Subscriptions: Phyllis Crittenden
Associate Director, Production: Johanna Harris
Executive Director, Global Publishing: Catherine Chopp Hinckley, MA, PhD

JOINT COMMISSION ENTERPRISE REVIEWERS

Jennifer Anderson, DNP, APRN, CNS
John Berry, RN, MSN
Karen E. Black, RN, BSN, MSHA, CPHQ
Andrea Browne, PhD, DABR
Robert Campbell, PharmD, BCSCP
Caroline Christensen, BS
Jeff Conway, MPH
Christina Cordero, PhD, MPH
Mark A. Crafton, MPA, MT(ASCP)
David Eickemeyer, MBA
Monnette Geronimo, MBA
Jenna Gillette, MHA, PMP
Kenneth J. Hébert Jr., MAOM, CHSP, CHEP
Debbie Holzer, RN, MSN, CRRN
Heather Hurley, BS
James Kendig, MS, CHSP, HEM
Karen Kolendra, RN, MSN, CPHQ
Ryan Kollereb, MBA, MPH
Chad Larson, MBA
Erin Lawler, MS, CPPS
Tim Markijohn, MBA\MHA, CHFM, CHE
Herman A. McKenzie, MBA, CHSP
Angela Murray, MSN, RN
Phavinee Thongkhong-Park, RN, PhD
Stacey Paul, MSN, RN, APN/PMHNP-BC
Kathryn Petrovic, MSN, RN-BC
Patrick Phelan, MBA
Natalya Rosenberg, PhD, RN
Thomas Todro, MBA, CBET
Cherie Ulaskas, MT(ASCP), MA
Kathy Valencia, MSN
Tabitha V. Vieweg, MBA, BSN, RN
John C. Wallin, MS, RN
Tiffany Wiksten, DNP, RN, CIC
Gina Zimmermann, MS

Table of Contents

Access to the Digital Tools in This Book

TOOLS

The tools in this book are available as downloadable, customizable resources that can be modified, shared, and/or distributed internally to staff in your health care organization.

To access these tools, visit bit.ly/4cm3Mx1. Users of the e-book can click on each tool title in the "Tool" feature.

Introduction

Welcome to the *Toolkit for New Accreditation Professionals*, Fourth Edition. The *Toolkit for New Accreditation Professionals* will introduce you to The Joint Commission and will lead accreditation professionals, like you, through the Joint Commission accreditation process—from the electronic application for accreditation (E-App) to the survey and accreditation decision and beyond into continuous compliance. This book introduces concepts critical to your position, with activities to get you started applying those concepts in your everyday responsibilities.

WHO SHOULD READ THIS BOOK?

Everyone. Obviously, if you are charged with monitoring and ensuring compliance with Joint Commission standards at your organization or department, this book is for you. But compliance is everyone's job. Health care leaders, clinical staff, environment of care specialists, building managers, and anyone else who does work to maintain and sustain compliance with Joint Commission requirements can benefit from the information and tools contained in this book.

WHY YOU NEED THIS BOOK

Becoming accredited and maintaining accreditation are immensely complex and cross-disciplinary endeavors. Accreditation has lots of moving parts. Each health care organization is different, of course, but this book serves as a primer for anyone who needs an overview of the accreditation process or who is responsible for a substantial part of it.

THE SCOPE OF THIS BOOK

This *Toolkit* is a guide to help you—an accreditation professional—better understand The Joint Commission and the many facets of the accreditation process and its requirements. In addition to offering accreditation, The Joint Commission has standalone and accreditation program-specific certifications for care and services provided for nearly any chronic disease or condition. The Joint Commission also offers other types of certification not connected to diseases or conditions such as healthcare sustainability and health care equity. The Joint Commission also offers one verification program for maternal levels of care. Although there are many similarities among the accreditation, certification, and verification processes, there also are many differences. This book focuses on the accreditation process. Although there is some discussion on Joint Commission certifications and verification, these discussions are included to tie them together with accreditation. We encourage you to visit The Joint Commission's website or contact your account executive for additional information—including eligibility requirements and the review process—on certification and verification programs your organization is interested in pursuing.

WHAT'S NEW IN THIS EDITION

In addition to updated resources and information, changes to the fourth edition of the *Toolkit* include the following new content:

- Top Challenging Standards at the beginning of applicable standards chapters in Part 4
- Test Your Knowledge quiz at the end of each chapter
- New sidebars on Joint Commission priorities (health care equity, sustainable healthcare, and workforce safety and well-being)
- Joint Commission and National Quality Forum strategic affiliation
- New certification and verification programs (Maternal Levels of Care Verification, Advanced Certification in Perinatal Care, Health Care Equity Certification, Sustainable Healthcare Certification, and Memory Care Certification)
- Evidence of Standards Compliance (ESC) tool (filled-out example)
- Patient safety topic portals
- Cybersecurity as it relates to records and information technology

Throughout this new edition, material previously included in the relevant chapters of the third edition has been moved to the appendices to minimize repetition and intrusion. For example, there is a "Recommended Resources" section that directs you to additional Joint Commission–related content, as well as other references to support you as you learn about or refresh your knowledge of these topics. Finally, the dozens of tools included in the *Toolkit* have been meticulously reviewed to ensure their accuracy and updated or replaced as applicable. This edition is accurate as of the publication date.

HOW THIS BOOK IS ORGANIZED

This new edition of the book is broken down into four parts:

- **Part 1: Understanding The Joint Commission.** Chapters 1 and 2. Covers the basics of The Joint Commission, its mission and vision, and the accreditation programs.
- **Part 2: Understanding the Accreditation Process.** Chapters 3–6. Provides an in-depth look at the process of obtaining and maintaining Joint Commission accreditation.
- **Part 3: Understanding Joint Commission–Related Data.** Chapters 7 and 8. Takes you on a deep dive into proven methods for working with performance measures and collecting, analyzing, and using meaningful data to drive compliance, improvement, and change.
- **Part 4: Understanding Challenging Standards.** Chapters 9–19. Focuses on and lists the major standards topics and provides a starting point for addressing challenging compliance areas. Each of these chapters includes "Key Concepts," which are important aspects of the relevant standards areas that will help you focus your thinking about compliance. The "Why Do I Need to Know This Now?" and "Where Do I Start?" features will help you tie concepts presented in each chapter to your real-world experience as an accreditation professional and provide direction for how to begin addressing concerns. Each of the standards-focused chapters includes a section on "Critical Challenges" to help you understand particularly challenging aspects of standards and/or elements of performance (EPs). And at the end of each chapter we have included tools we think you will find useful as you get started.

BOOK FEATURES

Each chapter includes the same types of features presented in the same order, so navigation is easy. And in the e-book version, internal links allow you to easily search for terms and navigate across chapters. (For example, terms that appear in the Glossary in the print version are shown in red text.)

Information is presented in clear, concise language in a colorful and easy-to-follow format that includes a variety of valuable features, including the following:

The Manual	→	Relevant *Comprehensive Accreditation Manual* chapters identified here are applicable to the content of the chapter.
The Big Idea	→	Presents the chapter theme/overview.
Key Concepts	→	Each chapter highlights 2–6 important ideas.
Why Do I Need to Know This Now?	→	Summarizes why each key concept is crucial to the safety of care recipients and accreditation success.
Where Do I Start?	→	Recommends practical activities for learning and applying the key concepts.
Critical Challenges	→	Gives an overview of challenging requirements across programs that have recently been most frequently cited by surveyors.
Picture This	→	Offers a visual presentation of a critical concept.
Just Imagine...	→	Provides a brief scenario that illustrates an important issue.
I Heard That...	→	Shares common standards-related "myths" and their rebuttals.
Priority	→	New sidebars detail Joint Commission priorities
Test Your Knowledge	→	Each chapter closes with a knowledge check.
Tools	→	Delivers downloadable, customizable tools.

TOOLS AND RESOURCES

The majority of the chapters include customizable tools. Near the end of the book is a section titled "Recommended Resources." The resources include links to further information on Joint Commission enterprise websites and government agency websites to help you address and understand the concepts discussed in the book.

LIST OF ACRONYMS

Throughout this book you will encounter commonly used acronyms pertaining to your job, health care, and the Joint Commission accreditation process. These include the abbreviations used to refer to The Joint Commission's hard-copy *Comprehensive Accreditation Manual* and manual chapters; the following is a quick reference for these terms:

Manual Title Acronym	Manual Title
CAMAC	*Comprehensive Accreditation Manual for Ambulatory Care*
CAMALC	*Comprehensive Accreditation Manual for Assisted Living Communities*
CAMBHC	*Comprehensive Accreditation Manual for Behavioral Health Care and Human Services*
CAMCAH	*Comprehensive Accreditation Manual for Critical Access Hospitals*
CAMH	*Comprehensive Accreditation Manual for Hospitals*
CAMHC	*Comprehensive Accreditation Manual for Home Care*
CAMLAB	*Comprehensive Accreditation Manual for Laboratory and Point-of-Care Testing*
CAMNCC	*Comprehensive Accreditation Manual for Nursing Care Centers*
CAMOBS	*Comprehensive Accreditation Manual for Office-Based Surgery Practices*

Chapter Title Acronym	Manual Chapter Title
ACC	The Accreditation Process
APR	Accreditation Participation Requirements
DC	Document and Process Control
EC	Environment of Care®
EM	Emergency Management
EQ	Equipment Management
ESP	Early Survey Policy
HR*	Human Resources
IC	Infection Prevention and Control
IM	Information Management
LD	Leadership
LS	Life Safety
MC	Medication Compounding
MM	Medication Management
MS	Medical Staff
NPSG	National Patient Safety Goals®
NR	Nursing
PC†	Provision of Care, Treatment, and Services
PCMH	Primary Care Medical Home Certification Option
PI	Performance Improvement
PM	Performance Measurement and the ORYX® Initiative

* In the *CAMBHC*, this chapter is titled "Human Resources Management" (HRM).
† In the *CAMBHC*, this chapter is titled "Care, Treatment, and Services" (CTS).

Chapter Title Acronym	Manual Chapter Title
PS[‡]	Patient Safety Systems
QR	The Joint Commission Quality Report
QSA	Quality System Assessment for Nonwaived Testing
RC	Record of Care, Treatment, and Services
RI	Rights and Responsibilities of the Individual
RWD	Required Written Documentation
SAG	Standards Applicability Grid
SE	Sentinel Event Policy
TS	Transplant Safety
WT	Waived Testing

JOINT COMMISSION REQUIREMENTS

Accreditation is achieved through compliance with Joint Commission standards, which are available to your organization through two distinct mediums. As an accreditation professional in your organization, you have complimentary access to E-dition® through your organization's secure *Joint Commission Connect®* extranet site. This complimentary access allows for one single user at a time in E-dition. E-dition provides access to the standards your organization is accredited under. Joint Commission Resources (JCR) also publishes a for-sale book or e-book version of the *Comprehensive Accreditation Manual* for most health care settings. JCR also sells software, specifically unlimited user access to E-dition as well as an assessment tool built on top of E-dition called Tracers with AMP. See the JCR website for more information about these for-sale options. Please note that it is not necessary to purchase these products to become or remain accredited. In addition, accreditation process information can be found on E-dition and in the book or e-book version of the manual. The standards and accreditation process information posted on E-dition and published in the book or e-book manuals are identical. Exceptions to this alignment include instances when there are interim releases to E-dition that do not fall into the regularly scheduled biannual (January 1 or July 1) releases or for book or e-book versions of manuals that are published once a year.

A WORD ABOUT TERMINOLOGY

The health care field is vast and provides care, treatment, and services to many individuals who may identify as a patient, an individual served, a resident, or a client. To respect this diverse field, the term *care recipient* has been used—as applicable—throughout the *Toolkit* to describe individuals who receive or have received care, treatment, and/or services.

---

‡ In the *CAMBHC*, this chapter is titled "Safety Systems for Individuals Served" (SSIS); in CAMALC, this chapter is titled "Resident Safety Systems" (RSS).

ACKNOWLEDGMENTS

JCR gratefully acknowledges the time and insights of the subject matter experts at The Joint Commission (listed on the copyright page). We would also like to thank our reviewer, O. Denise Wilson, DNP, RN, CPPS, CJCP, HACP, System Director, Regulatory Compliance, Accreditation, and Complaints/Grievances, Center for Clinical Excellence (CCE), SSM Health.

PART 1
Understanding The Joint Commission

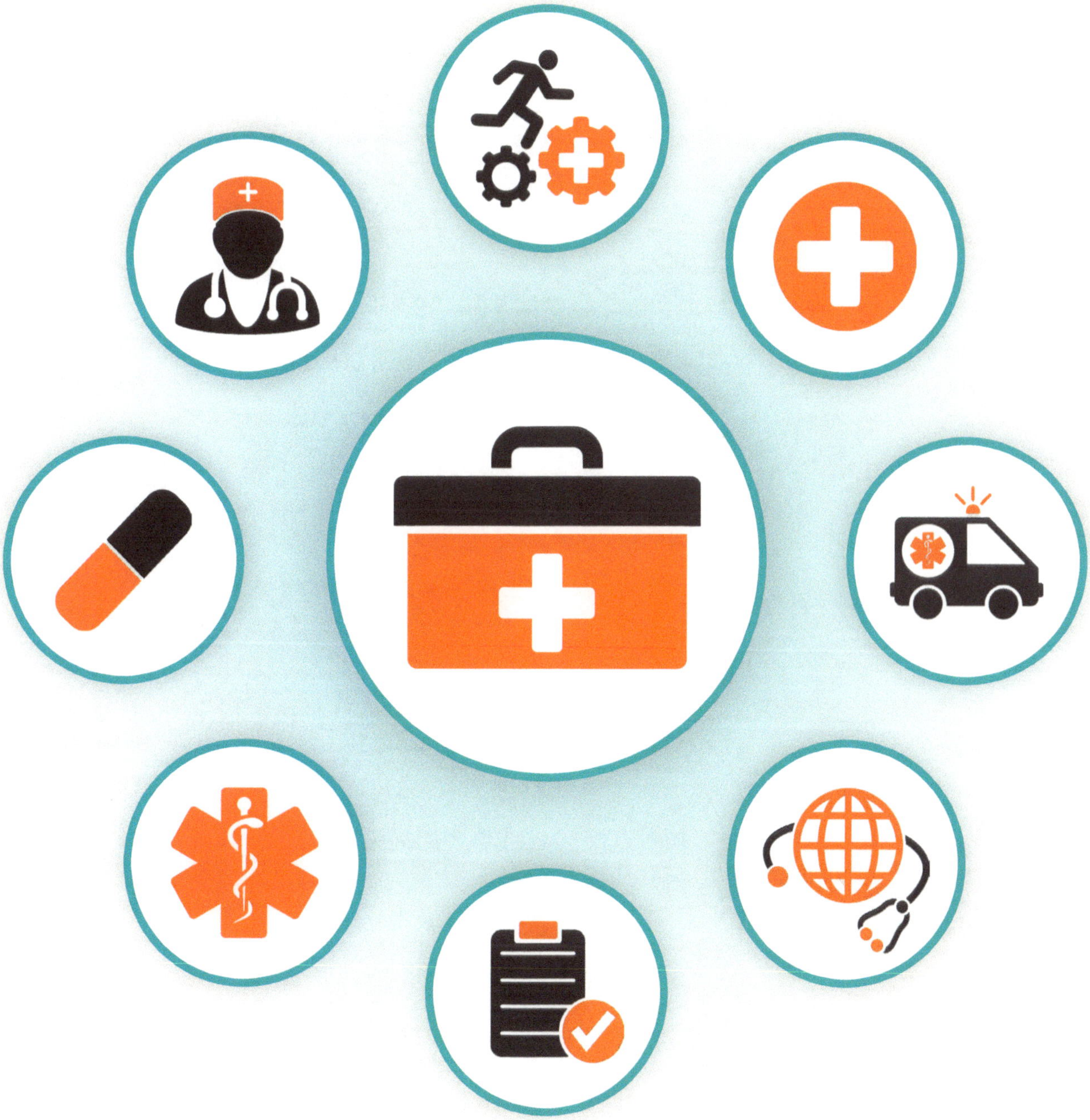

About The Joint Commission

CHAPTER 1

THE BIG IDEA

The Joint Commission is an independent not-for-profit organization that accredits and certifies more than 22,000 health care organizations in the United States. Joint Commission accreditation, certification, and verification are marks of quality and commitment to meeting certain standards of quality and performance. The Joint Commission is your partner in safety and quality across the continuum of care.

KEY CONCEPTS

- What Is The Joint Commission Enterprise?
- Your Partner in Safety and Quality

THE MANUAL

Following are the relevant Joint Commission E-dition® or *Comprehensive Accreditation Manual* chapters:

- "Introduction: How Joint Commission Accreditation Can Help on the Road to High Reliability" (INTRO)
- "Patient Safety Systems" (PS) [not assisted living community or behavioral health care and human services]
- "Resident Safety Systems" (RSS) [assisted living community only]
- "Safety Systems for Individuals Served" (SSIS) [behavioral health care and human services only]
- "Sentinel Event Policy" (SE)

KEY CONCEPT

WHAT IS THE JOINT COMMISSION ENTERPRISE?

The Joint Commission enterprise is an umbrella term that refers to The Joint Commission itself and its ancillary bodies, including Joint Commission Resources (JCR), Joint Commission International (JCI), and the National Quality Forum (NQF). Together, these companies make up the "enterprise," with The Joint Commission as the head.

THE JOINT COMMISSION'S MISSION AND VISION

Mission: To continuously improve health care for the public, in collaboration with other stakeholders, by evaluating health care organizations and inspiring them to excel in providing safe and effective care of the highest quality and value.

Vision: All people always experience the safest, highest-quality, best-value health care across all settings.

The Joint Commission

The Joint Commission seeks to improve the safety and quality of health care by offering accreditation to health care organizations and certification and verification to health care programs. The Joint Commission sets quality standards, evaluates organizational performance through surveys, and advances safety and quality of care provided to all care recipients.

Joint Commission Resources

JCR is a global, knowledge-based organization that provides innovative solutions designed to help health care organizations improve the safety and quality of health care to all care recipients. An affiliate of The Joint Commission, JCR provides expertise on the many issues organizations face in a challenging health care environment through a variety of products and services, including education programs, publications and e-products, and health care consulting and custom education. JCR is dedicated to helping health care organizations worldwide improve the quality and safety of their care, treatment, and services.

Joint Commission International

JCI extends The Joint Commission's mission worldwide by assisting international health care organizations, public health agencies, health ministries, and others to improve the quality and safety of health care to all individuals. Established in 1994 as a division of JCR, JCI's accreditation program was developed by international experts and sets uniform, achievable expectations for structures, processes, and outcomes for health care organizations. JCI offers accreditation for different types of health care organizations and certification for treatment of specific disease, condition, or clinical care services in more than 70 countries.

National Quality Forum

In August 2023 The Joint Commission and National Quality Forum (NQF) announced a strategic affiliation to accelerate improvements in health for all people.

Established in 1999, NQF works with members of the health care community to drive measurable health improvements together. NQF is a not-for-profit, membership-based organization that gives all health care stakeholders a voice in advancing quality measures and improvement strategies that lead to better outcomes and greater value.

NQF joined The Joint Commission enterprise while maintaining its independence in convening and developing consensus-based measures, implementation guidance, and practices that benefit all stakeholders. This allows both The Joint Commission and NQF to build on their shared expertise in measuring quality and rationalizing the measurement landscape so the focus shifts to advancing key outcomes. Notably, NQF continues to focus on accelerating widespread use of high-impact, low-burden measures that achieve affordable improvements in health for all.

The affiliation bolsters The Joint Commission's national and international processes in evidence-based, data-driven, and outcomes-oriented accreditation, certification, and verification, thereby accelerating improvements across the continuum of care while reducing the burden of measurement on health care organizations and workers.

WHY DO I NEED TO KNOW THIS NOW?

The Joint Commission is more than an accrediting body that comes to your organization once every three years to evaluate your safety and quality processes. The enterprise provides a wealth of information, resources, and support to help you maintain a safe, high-quality environment and tackle challenges you face.

WHERE DO I START?

- **Research.** Visit the various Joint Commission websites to become familiar with the products and resources available to your organization. The "Recommended Resources" at the end of this book provides specific links to Joint Commission enterprise websites.

KEY CONCEPT

YOUR PARTNER IN SAFETY AND QUALITY

The Joint Commission is a global driver of quality improvement and patient safety in health care. The Joint Commission is your partner in safety and quality. Through leading practices, unmatched knowledge and expertise, and rigorous standards, we help organizations across the continuum of care lead the way to zero harm.

Surveys as Learning Opportunities

Think of each survey as a collaborative assessment of the organization's performance. It is an opportunity for the organization and its leaders to learn what the organization is doing well and identify where there is room for improvement. Sometimes these things are harder to see for those working within an organization, so it can be very useful to have an extra set of eyes take a look at your operations and give you an objective assessment of how well you are complying with standards, providing care and treatment to the population(s) you serve, reducing the potential for harm, and increasing reliability. Use your surveyors as the expert resource they are.

Sentinel Event Reporting

A sentinel event is a patient safety event (not primarily related to the natural course of a care recipient's illness or underlying condition) that reaches an individual and results in any of the following:

- death,
- severe harm (regardless of duration of harm), or
- permanent harm (regardless of severity of harm).

Sentinel events are a subcategory of adverse events.

Although organizations are not required to report sentinel events to The Joint Commission, accredited organizations must have a policy detailing how the organization addresses sentinel events. The specific requirements of that policy are included in the "Leadership" (LD), "Performance Improvement" (PI), and "Sentinel Event Policy" (SE) chapters of E-dition or the *Comprehensive Accreditation Manual*. The organization must complete a thorough comprehensive systematic analysis (most commonly a root cause analysis) to determine why the event occurred. The organization must then create a corrective action plan to prevent similar events from happening, implement the plan, and monitor its effectiveness.

There is no penalty for not reporting sentinel events to The Joint Commission, but organizations are strongly encouraged to do so. Self-reporting reinforces the organization's message to the public that it is doing everything it can to prevent a recurrence. Sharing information, particularly lessons learned, with The Joint Commission enhances The Joint Commission's Sentinel Event Database, which may help other organizations prevent similar events. Also, contacting The Joint Commission following a sentinel event allows you to avail yourself of the wealth of expertise and experience of its staff. They can help you analyze root causes, redesign processes, monitor performance improvement practices, and other aspects of the sentinel event process.

Twice a year via *Joint Commission Perspectives*®, the official monthly newsletter of The Joint Commission, The Joint Commission releases data on sentinel events. This information may help performance improvement professionals identify areas for improvement in their organizations. The more organizations report their own sentinel events, the better and more meaningful sentinel event statistics become. The Joint Commission sentinel event data not only identify the relative frequency of different categories of sentinel events reported each year but also provide information on trends in the occurrence of the most commonly reported sentinel event categories.

Reported Sentinel Event—Falls

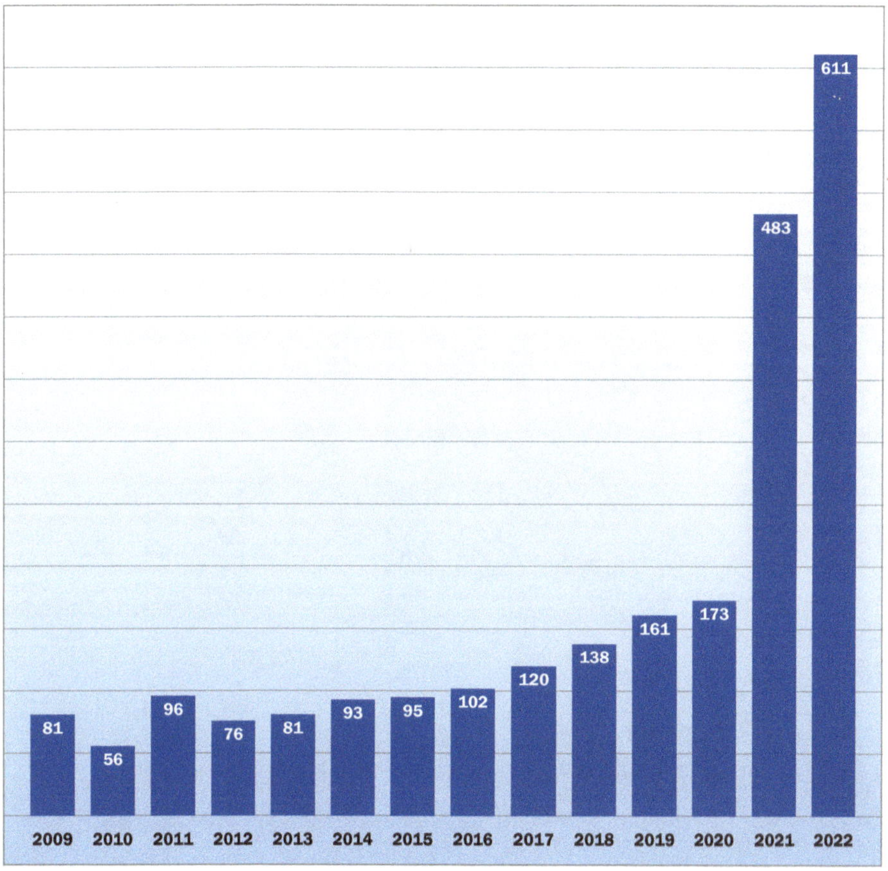

In the past few years, The Joint Commission reviewed more than 1,000 patient falls. Any individual—staff, care recipient, visitor—can be harmed by falling in any type of health care facility. To help health care organizations determine if a fall qualifies as a sentinel event, The Joint Commission includes a definition for fall event in its Sentinel Event Policy.

WHY DO I NEED TO KNOW THIS NOW?

Knowing what The Joint Commission is and what its role is in helping you and your organization provide safe and high-quality care, treatment, and services to all care recipients will help you as you acclimate to your new role as an accreditation professional in health care.

WHERE DO I START?

- **Connect with The Joint Commission.** Visit and bookmark the various Joint Commission websites (see "Recommended Resources" near the back of this book). There are numerous resources and links available to help you know The Joint Commission and the other entities that make up the enterprise.

- **Reach out to your account executive.** Whether you are brand new to accreditation or new to your organization as well as accreditation, the account executive assigned to your organization can provide valuable insight as you learn about your role.
- **Immerse yourself.** This book is a great start! Beyond this title, however, you should familiarize yourself with your organization's secure *Joint Commission Connect®* extranet site and E-dition or the *Comprehensive Accreditation Manual*(s).

Test Your Knowledge

1. Which of the following are part of The Joint Commission enterprise? (Select all that apply.)
   - ☐ a. Accreditation Commission for Health Care
   - ☐ b. Joint Commission International
   - ☐ c. Joint Commission Resources
   - ☐ d. National Quality Forum
2. Which of the following is the mission of The Joint Commission?
   - ☐ a. To improve the quality and safety of health care
   - ☐ b. To facilitate government reimbursement
   - ☐ c. To reduce redundancy between external agencies
3. What is the mission of Joint Commission Resources?
   - ☐ a. To provide education, publications, software, and technical assistance to improve the quality and safety of health care
   - ☐ b. To develop standards to assess organizations' delivery of care
   - ☐ c. To be The Joint Commission enterprise's start-up incubator
4. What is the purpose of Joint Commission International? (Select all that apply.)
   - ☐ a. To provide solutions to improve the quality and safety of international health care
   - ☐ b. To evaluate an organization's quality and safety
   - ☐ c. To reduce redundancy between government agencies
   - ☐ d. To develop new products and services
5. Which of the following describes the purpose of a Joint Commission survey?
   - ☐ a. To educate staff and leadership and assess the organization's compliance with Joint Commission standards
   - ☐ b. To validate the organization's compliance with Joint Commission policies and procedures and inform leadership about high reliability
   - ☐ c. To provide information and determine the quality of sentinel event corrective actions

(continued)

6. Which of the following statements about sentinel events is true?
   - ☐ a. All patient harm events are considered sentinel events.
   - ☐ b. Any sentinel event must be reported to The Joint Commission.
   - ☐ c. All patient harm events require a root cause analysis.
   - ☐ d. Sentinel events identified by your organization are voluntarily reported to The Joint Commission.
7. A provider informs you that they inadvertently performed a skin biopsy on the wrong patient earlier in the week. There was no serious injury, and eventually the right patient received the procedure. This event ______________.
   - ☐ a. would be considered a sentinel event
   - ☐ b. must be reported
   - ☐ c. requires a report to your chief executive officer
   - ☐ d. would be identified by a survey
8. Which of the following would be the best person in The Joint Commission enterprise to assist you with any questions about your organization's accreditation?
   - ☐ a. Standards Interpretation Group staff
   - ☐ b. Your account executive
   - ☐ c. Continuous Survey Readiness consultant
   - ☐ d. Chief executive officer

Understanding Joint Commission Accreditation, Certification, and Verification

CHAPTER 2

THE BIG IDEA

What exactly are Joint Commission accreditation, certification, and verification? Accreditation, certification, and verification are designations conferred by The Joint Commission that symbolize a health care organization's commitment to meeting rigorous standards of quality and safety for the populations it serves. Achieving accreditation, certification, and/or verification requires collaboration between organization and Joint Commission staff throughout the entire process—from completing the application through the survey or review and follow-up activities. Accreditation, certification, and verification have several benefits for the organization, including improved quality and safety and increased community confidence.

KEY CONCEPTS

- What Are Joint Commission Accreditation, Certification, and Verification?
- Eligibility Requirements

THE MANUAL

Following are the relevant Joint Commission E-dition® or *Comprehensive Accreditation Manual* chapters:

- "The Accreditation Process" (ACC)
- "Introduction: How Joint Commission Accreditation Can Help on the Road to High Reliability" (INTRO)

KEY CONCEPT

WHAT ARE JOINT COMMISSION ACCREDITATION, CERTIFICATION, AND VERIFICATION?

Accreditation is the seal of approval given by The Joint Commission to entire health care organizations. It is a mark of quality that attests to the organization's compliance with Joint Commission standards and commitment to excellence.

The Joint Commission also offers certification to programs within health care organizations that meet more rigorous program-specific guidelines based on research and industry best practices.

In addition, The Joint Commission offers a verification review, which assesses an organization's capabilities to provide care appropriate for a care recipient's condition.

Benefits of Joint Commission Accreditation, Certification, and Verification

Why should you work to become accredited, certified, and/or verified? The following list of benefits outline what you and your organization gain by achieving and maintaining Joint Commission accreditation, as well as the benefits of certification and verification if your organization chooses to pursue those options.

- **Benefits of Joint Commission Accreditation**
  - **Helps organize and strengthen safety efforts.** Safety and quality of care issues for all care recipients are at the forefront of Joint Commission standards and initiatives.
  - **Strengthens community confidence in the quality and safety of care, treatment, and services.** Achieving accreditation makes a strong statement to the community about an organization's efforts to provide the highest-quality services.
  - **Provides a competitive edge in the marketplace.** Accreditation may provide a marketing advantage in a competitive health care environment and improve the ability to secure new business.
  - **Improves risk management and risk reduction.** Joint Commission standards focus on state-of-the-art performance improvement strategies that help health care organizations continuously improve the safety and quality of care, which can reduce the risk of error or low-quality care.
  - **Reduces liability insurance costs.** By enhancing risk management efforts, accreditation may improve access to and reduce the cost of liability insurance coverage.
  - **Provides professional advice and counsel, enhancing staff education.** Joint Commission surveyors are experienced health care professionals trained to provide expert advice and education during the survey.
  - **Provides a customized, intensive review.** Joint Commission surveyors come from a variety of health care industries and are assigned to organizations

that match their background. The standards also are specific to each accreditation program, so each survey is relevant to your industry.

- **Enhances staff recruitment and development.** An organization that is Joint Commission accredited can attract more highly qualified personnel, who prefer to serve in an accredited organization. Accredited organizations also provide additional opportunities for staff to develop their skills and knowledge about quality and safety.
- **Provides deeming authority for regulatory certifications.** Some accredited health care organizations qualify for Medicare and Medicaid certification (including hospitals, critical access hospitals, advanced diagnostic imaging suppliers, and suppliers of durable medical equipment, prosthetics, orthotics, and supplies) without undergoing a separate government quality inspection, which eases the burdens of duplicative federal and state regulatory agency surveys. Opioid treatment programs accredited under The Joint Commission's Behavioral Health Care and Human Services (BHC) program are afforded deemed status by the US Substance Abuse and Mental Health Services Administration (SAMHSA).
- **Fulfills regulatory requirements in select states.** Laws may require certain health care providers to acquire accreditation for their organization. Those organizations already accredited by The Joint Commission may be compliant and need not undergo any additional surveys or inspections.
- **Recognized by insurers and other third parties.** In some markets, accreditation is becoming a prerequisite to eligibility for insurance reimbursement and for participation in managed care plans or contract bidding.
- **Provides a framework for organizational structure and management.** Accreditation involves maintaining a high level of quality and compliance with the latest standards and being ready for survey at any time. Joint Commission standards offer a framework for organizational structure, based on best practices, within which each organization can tailor a structure to fit the needs of its care recipients.
- **Aligns health care organizations with one of the most respected names in health care.** The Joint Commission is widely recognized by health care providers, policy makers, educators, and other key stakeholders as the preeminent standards-setting and accrediting organization in health care. Being accredited by The Joint Commission demonstrates an organization's commitment to the highest standards for safety and quality.

Benefits of Joint Commission Certification

- **Improves the quality of care by reducing variation in clinical processes.** The Joint Commission's standards and emphasis on following clinical practice guidelines help organizations establish a consistent approach to care, reducing the risk of error.
- **Provides a framework for program structure and management.** Certification standards help organize the management of the program. This helps to maintain a consistently high level of quality, using effective data-driven performance improvement.
- **Provides an objective assessment of clinical excellence.** Joint Commission reviewers have significant experience working in the field and

in evaluating disease-specific care and other certification programs. They can provide expert advice and education on good practices during the review.

- **Creates a loyal, cohesive clinical team.** Certification provides an opportunity for staff to develop their skills and knowledge. Achieving certification provides the clinical team with common goals and a concrete validation of their combined efforts.
- **Promotes a culture of excellence across the organization.** Consistent alignment with Joint Commission certification standards promotes an environment of continuous improvement for the care of individuals.
- **Facilitates marketing, contracting, and reimbursement.** Certification may provide an advantage in a competitive health care marketplace and improve the ability to secure new business.
- **Strengthens community confidence in the quality and safety of care, treatment, and services.** Achieving and displaying The Joint Commission's Gold Seal of Approval® makes a strong statement to the community about an organization's commitment to providing the highest-quality services.
- **Fulfills regulatory requirements in select states.** Certification may meet certain regulatory requirements in some states, which can reduce duplication on the part of certified organizations.

Benefits of Joint Commission Verification

- **Helps assure stakeholders.** Verification indicates that providers have the clinical capabilities and expertise to safely provide the services they offer.
- **Facilitates collaboration.** Verification standards help high-risk patients get routed to facilities equipped to handle complex or emergent patient conditions.

WHY DO I NEED TO KNOW THIS NOW?

You and your organization will invest a good amount of time and resources to achieve and maintain accreditation, certification, and/or verification. It's important to know what the return on that investment will be. Achieving accreditation is a benefit itself, but having strong, functional processes in place and cultivating a safe culture for your organization will better support your goal to provide safe, high-quality care, treatment, and services.

WHERE DO I START?

- **Immerse yourself.** As you acclimate to your new role, learn what the needs of your organization are by reviewing past and ongoing performance improvement activities. If your organization is already accredited by The Joint Commission, look back at previous survey/review activities.

PICTURE THIS

Joint Commission Accreditation, Certification, and Verification Programs

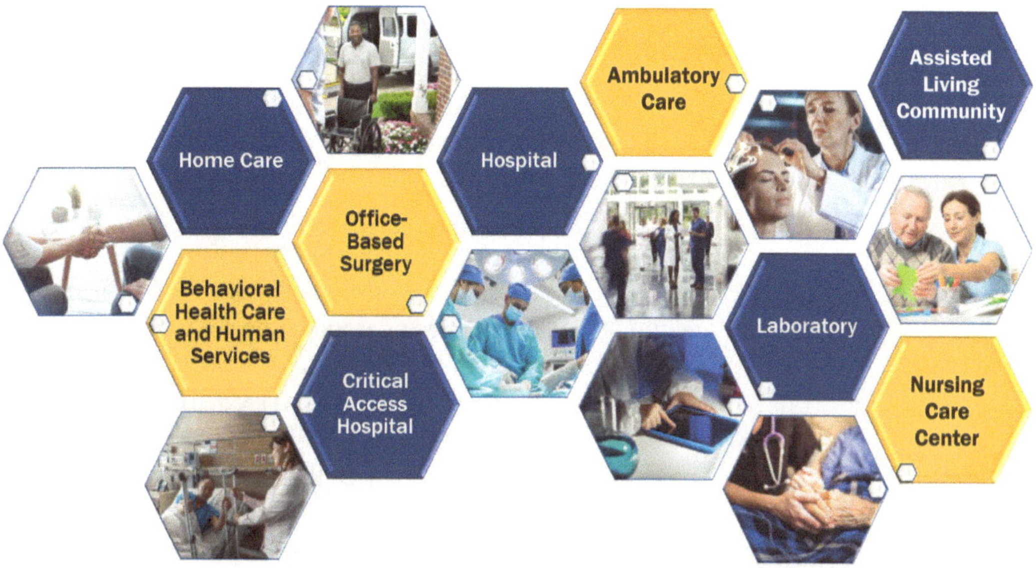

Ambulatory Care Certifications

- Advanced Total Hip and Total Knee Replacement
- Integrated Care
- Primary Care Medical Home

Nursing Care Center Certifications

- Core Disease-Specific Care
- Integrated Care
- Memory Care
- Post-Acute Care

Behavioral Health Care and Human Services Certifications

- Behavioral Health Home
- Certified Community Behavioral Health Clinic
- Core Disease-Specific Care
- Integrated Care
- Opioid Treatment Program

Assisted Living Community Certification

- Memory Care

Home Care Certifications

- Community-Based Palliative Care
- Core Disease-Specific Care
- Integrated Care

Hospital Certifications

- Cardiac
- Orthopedic
- Stroke
- Health Care Equity
- Responsible Use of Health Data
- Sustainable Healthcare
- Disease-Specific Care, including joint replacement, spine surgery, and stroke care
- Medication Compounding
- Advanced Perinatal Care
- Palliative Care
- Patient Blood Management
- Primary Care Medical Home
- Pathways and Structures Helping Leaders Advance Quality
- Payor Recognitions

Hospital Verification

- Maternal Levels of Care

The Joint Commission currently offers accreditation for nine program settings, a variety of certifications, and one verification program; two new accreditation programs will be introduced in 2024: Telehealth and Rural Health Clinic.

KEY CONCEPT

ELIGIBILITY REQUIREMENTS

The following list provides basic eligibility requirements for health care organizations seeking accreditation. For requirements specific to your program setting, see "The Accreditation Process" (ACC) chapter on E-dition or in your book or e-book version of the *Comprehensive Accreditation Manual*.

- The organization is in the United States or its territories; if outside the United States, the organization is operated by the US government or under a charter of the US Congress.
- If required by law, the organization has a facility license or registration to conduct its scope of services.
- The organization can demonstrate that it continually assesses and improves the quality of its care, treatment, and/or services. This process includes a review by clinicians, including those knowledgeable in the type of care, treatment, and/or services provided at the organization.
- The organization identifies the services it provides, indicating which care, treatment, and/or services it provides directly, under contract, or through some other arrangement.
- The organization provides services that can be evaluated by Joint Commission standards.
- The tests, treatments, or interventions provided at the organization are prescribed or ordered by a licensed practitioner in accordance with state and federal requirements.

WHY DO I NEED TO KNOW THIS NOW?

To be proficient in your role, you need to know the ins and outs of Joint Commission accreditation and, as applicable to your organization, certification, and verification. The more you know about the process and expectations, the better grasp you will have on managing survey readiness initiatives.

WHERE DO I START?

- **Familiarize yourself with E-dition and/or your *Comprehensive Accreditation Manual*.** All the requirements that surveyors will be evaluating are on E-dition or in the manual. These two resources include general information about the accreditation process as well as program-specific eligibility requirements.

Test Your Knowledge

1. Which of the following describes Joint Commission accreditation?
   - ☐ a. An award to an organization for meeting Joint Commission requirements
   - ☐ b. A survey of your health care organization
   - ☐ c. Recognition granted by the Centers for Medicare & Medicaid Services
   - ☐ d. The recommendation given upon completion of a survey

2. Which of the following describes Joint Commission disease-specific certification?
   - ☐ a. Recognition for providing patient-condition specific care
   - ☐ b. The onsite review of your health care organization
   - ☐ c. Recognition granted by the Centers for Medicare & Medicaid Services
   - ☐ d. The certificate granted to an organization for completing the accreditation process

3. Which of the following is not an eligibility requirement for a US organization to be Joint Commission accredited?
   - ☐ a. The organization is in the United States or its territories.
   - ☐ b. The organization is a nonprofit.
   - ☐ c. The organization provides services that can be evaluated by Joint Commission standards.
   - ☐ d. The organization can demonstrate that it continually assesses and improves the quality of its care, treatment, and services.

4. Which of the following are not eligible for Joint Commission accreditation? (Select all that apply.)
   - ☐ a. Ambulances
   - ☐ b. Medical air transport
   - ☐ c. Individual physicians, nurses, or other clinicians of your health care organization
   - ☐ d. A clinic physically separate from a hospital

5. Which of the following is not a benefit of Joint Commission accreditation?
   - ☐ a. Fulfills regulatory requirements in select states
   - ☐ b. Guarantees that an organization will no longer encounter any challenges
   - ☐ c. Helps organize and strengthen safety efforts
   - ☐ d. Reduces liability insurance costs

PART 2
Understanding the Accreditation Process

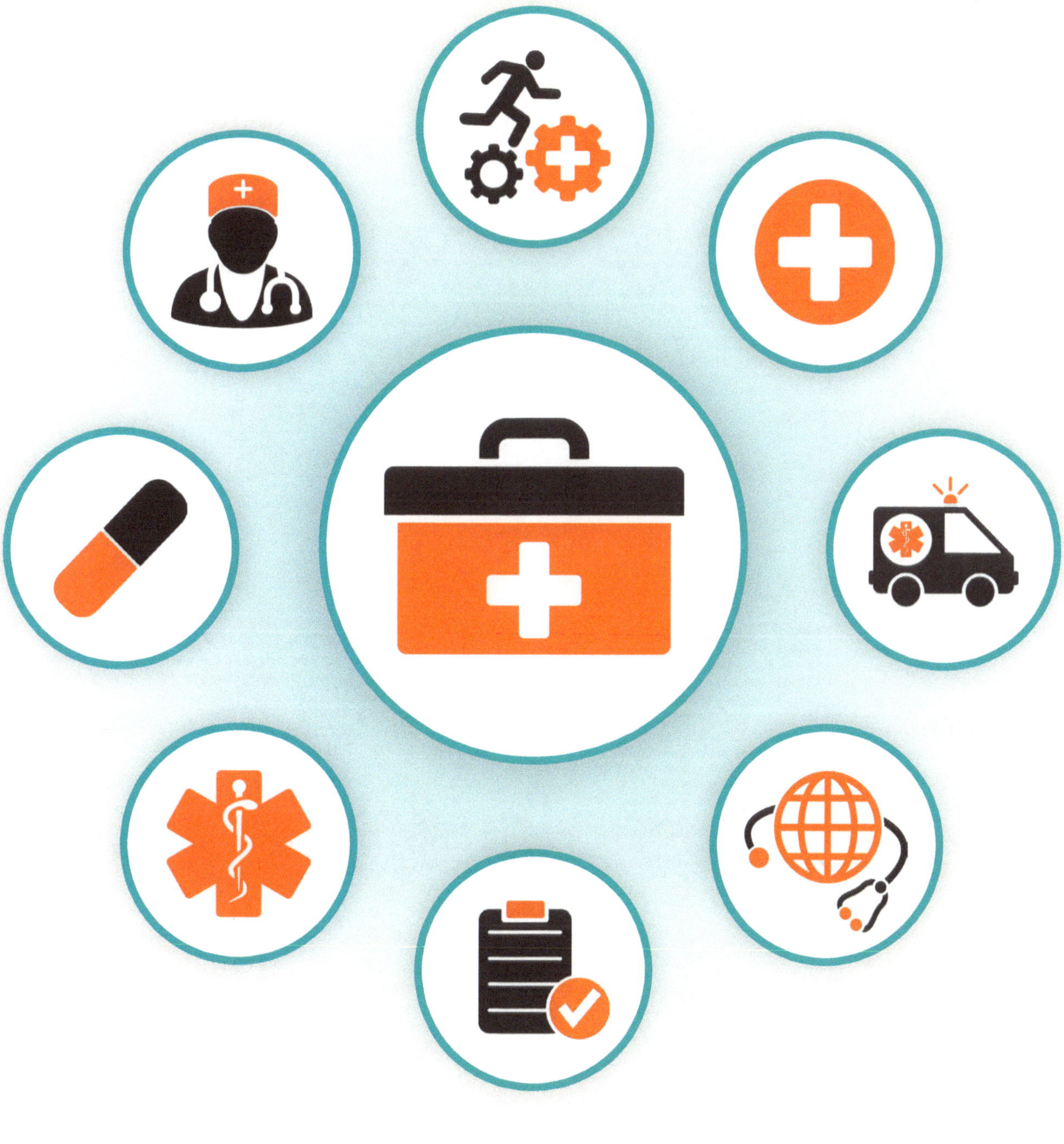

Preparing for an Accreditation Survey

CHAPTER 3

THE BIG IDEA

Joint Commission accreditation reflects a health care organization's ongoing commitment to the quality of care it provides to recipients of that care. An accreditation professional plays a vital role in guiding the organization through the accreditation process, central to obtaining and maintaining accreditation. Proper preparation for the survey is critical to success. In this chapter we will discuss areas to focus on as you get ready for your survey.

KEY CONCEPTS

- The First Steps
- Getting Started
- Working with Standards
- Survey Readiness

THE MANUAL

Following are the relevant Joint Commission E-dition® or *Comprehensive Accreditation Manual* chapters:

- "The Accreditation Process" (ACC)
- "Early Survey Policy" (ESP)

KEY CONCEPT

THE FIRST STEPS

The Joint Commission accredits thousands of health care organizations nationwide. If you're not currently one of those, you'll need to apply. If your organization is already accredited, you need to keep your accreditation information up to date in the electronic application for accreditation (E-App). Applying and updating are both done via your organization's *Joint Commission Connect*® extranet site.

Who Can Apply?

Broadly speaking, health care organizations in the United States, or those operated by the US government in other countries, that are licensed to provide their scope of services, provide services that can be evaluated by Joint Commission standards, and can demonstrate a commitment to improving their performance may apply for accreditation. Those seeking deemed status from the US Centers for Medicare & Medicaid Services (CMS), US Substance Abuse and Mental Health Services Administration (SAMHSA), or other deeming authorities must meet a set of requirements, such as Conditions of Participation (CoPs), Conditions for Coverage (CfCs), or other applicable requirements. The Joint Commission has deeming authority from CMS for certain types of health care organizations such as hospitals; therefore, being accredited by The Joint Commission means that that health care organization also meets CMS requirements and is therefore eligible for Medicare and Medicaid reimbursements.

Joint Commission Connect

Joint Commission Connect is a secure extranet website intended only for organizations accredited or certified or those seeking accreditation, certification, and/or verification by The Joint Commission. It is the primary way that The Joint Commission communicates with accredited, certified, and verified organizations. It contains many useful resources about the survey process and tools for continuous compliance, as well as your access to Joint Commission standards through E-dition. This site also allows you to exchange important and confidential information with The Joint Commission.

Each organization is responsible for designating who has access to the *Joint Commission Connect* extranet site. As an accreditation professional, you should have full access to *Joint Commission Connect*. Although only a select few in your organization also may have full access to the extranet site, limited access can be granted to staff, allowing them to access and use resources provided, such as E-dition and *Joint Commission Perspectives*®, without displaying confidential information. If you're an accredited organization, or an organization seeking Joint Commission accreditation, you can contact your account executive for access assistance.

WHY DO I NEED TO KNOW THIS NOW?

Every journey has a beginning. The journey to become Joint Commission accredited, certified, or verified is no different. If your organization is already accredited, certified, or verified, then your journey begins by understanding what is required by The Joint Commission and where to find that information.

WHERE DO I START?

- **Learn more.** The Joint Commission's website and your organization's *Joint Commission Connect* extranet site have many resources to guide you through various stages of the accreditation process.

KEY CONCEPT

GETTING STARTED

To begin the process of becoming accredited, certified, or verified by The Joint Commission, you will need to apply by completing the E-App. Familiarize yourself with your *Joint Commission Connect* extranet site to know how best to communicate with The Joint Commission and to use the resources provided to you as you prepare for your initial survey.

TOOL

E-App Checklist

The E-App

You can find the E-App under the **Survey Process** tab on your *Joint Commission Connect* extranet site. A video tutorial is available to help you navigate the application.

Note that the E-App isn't just for first-time applicants. It's also used to keep The Joint Commission informed of organizational changes throughout the year. You must update your E-App within 30 calendar days of a relevant change. Refer to "The Accreditation Process" (ACC) chapter on E-dition or the *Comprehensive Accreditation Manual* for a list of such changes.

Your Account Executive

After completing your E-App, you'll be assigned a dedicated account executive. This person serves as the primary contact between your organization and The Joint Commission. Your account executive coordinates survey planning and handles policies, procedures, accreditation/certification issues or services, and inquiries throughout the accreditation/certification/verification cycle. Your account executive is your go-to, a starred favorite on your help line, and your partner at The Joint Commission.

Early Survey Process

Early survey is an option for organizations not yet fully functioning that are seeking accreditation for the first time and want to start the accreditation process before providing care or meeting full eligibility criteria. It also allows an organization to validate that the foundational quality and safety concepts are in place before undergoing a full survey. The early survey process includes the following two surveys:

- **First Survey.** This survey is announced and limited in scope. It focuses on a discrete set of standards addressing primarily physical facilities, policies, and related structural issues. If those standards are met, the organization is granted Limited, Temporary Accreditation status. (This status isn't recognized by CMS.) If the standards aren't met, the organization must reapply and start the process over again. The standards assessed in this survey are listed in the "Early Survey Policy" (ESP) chapter on E-dition or in your *Comprehensive Accreditation Manual*.
- **Second Survey.** The second survey is a full, unannounced, initial accreditation survey. It's conducted for organizations that have been granted Limited, Temporary Accreditation status. The result of the second survey can be any of the full range of accreditation decisions. (See "Accreditation Outcomes" in Chapter 5 for more information.)

For organizations that choose the Early Survey option, it must be declared during the application process.

Deemed Status

What if you could cut down on the number of surveys you need to go through? You can, if you're deemed.

What is CMS? The Centers for Medicare & Medicaid Services (CMS) was founded in 1965 as a federal agency within the US Department of Health and Human Services to administer the Medicare and Medicaid programs. Medicare is a health insurance program for the elderly, and Medicaid is a health insurance program for those with limited income.

What it means to be deemed. Accreditation from The Joint Commission can often be used to meet certification standards for CMS, SAMHSA, and other regulatory authorities. It's known as deemed status or deeming. This is possible because the standards and elements of performance (EPs) required for Joint Commission accreditation meet or exceed the deeming organization's requirements. For example, CMS refers to its requirements as Conditions of Participation (CoPs) or Conditions for Coverage (CfCs).

"I heard that...

there are two separate sets of requirements we have to meet: one for Joint Commission accreditation and one for deemed status."

fact:

If your organization complies with Joint Commission accreditation standards, it meets or exceeds the standards required by the regulatory organization.

It's optional. Pursuing a deemed status survey with The Joint Commission is optional and, in fact, does not guarantee that an additional survey from a state agency may not be conducted. You still can undergo a survey from a state agency for regulatory certification.

Deemed status standards. Some standards and EPs listed on E-dition or in the *Comprehensive Accreditation Manual* are required *only* for organizations seeking to use Joint Commission accreditation for deemed status purposes. On E-dition, you can search for the term *deem* or *deemed* to identify these requirements; in the book or e-book version of the manual, these are always clearly marked in the standards, in boldface.

No guarantees. Where regulatory authorities have allowed, complying with Joint Commission standards and EPs will qualify your organization for deemed status. However, be aware that compliance with regulatory requirements doesn't guarantee compliance with Joint Commission accreditation standards. Why not? Because some Joint Commission standards don't directly link to requirements set by regulatory authorities and are above and beyond what may be required by CMS or others. For a side-by-side comparison of standards and regulatory requirements for settings with deeming, refer to the crosswalks on E-dition.

WHY DO I NEED TO KNOW THIS NOW?

Completing the application is the first step of the journey toward accreditation. In addition, if your organization is deemed or is considering becoming deemed, it will affect nearly all your accreditation activities.

WHERE DO I START?

- **Organize information:** Before you begin the application, gather the materials and information you'll need. The following are examples of information you may need to complete the application:
  - "Ready date" time frame
  - Employer identification number
  - CMS Certification Number (CCN), if applicable
  - Site demographic information, such as site name, address, and services provided
  - For each site, gather the following information as it is applicable to your setting and organization:
    - Annual patient visits/annual total of individuals served, average daily census, annual case volume
    - Number of licensed practitioners
    - Number of licensed clinical staff
    - Number of full-time staff
    - Hours of operation
    - List of services provided
- **Learn more.** The relationship of regulatory and Joint Commission requirements is one you should study before deciding to pursue or maintain deemed status.
- **Work with leaders.** Determine if your organization is or will be seeking deemed status. If you aren't already deemed, you'll need to lay out the prospect to your governing board or senior leaders. When your organization has decided (yea or nay), include this information in your E-App.

KEY CONCEPT

WORKING WITH STANDARDS

Joint Commission standards form the basis of an objective evaluation that can help organizations measure, assess, and improve performance. They are focused on important functions that are essential to delivering safe, high-quality care, treatment, and services.

General Overview of Joint Commission Standards

For each health care setting in which The Joint Commission accredits organizations, Joint Commission Resources (JCR), the official publisher of The Joint Commission, publishes E-dition (and in most programs a book or e-book version of the *Comprehensive Accreditation Manual*) that contains all the standards that apply to organizations in that setting. The standards are grouped into accreditation requirement chapters that correspond to the areas of activity on which your organization will be evaluated:

- Accreditation Participation Requirements (APR)
- Care, Treatment, and Services (CTS) [behavioral health care and human services only]
- Document and Process Control (DC) [laboratory only]
- Environment of Care (EC)
- Emergency Management (EM)
- Equipment, Devices, and Connectivity (EDC) [telehealth only]
- Equipment Management (EQ) [home care only]
- Human Resources (HR) [not behavioral health care and human services]
- Human Resources Management (HRM) [behavioral health care and human services only]
- Infection Prevention and Control (IC)
- Information Management (IM)
- Leadership (LD)
- Life Safety (LS) [not laboratory]
- Medical Staff (MS) [critical access hospitals and hospitals only]
- Medication Compounding (MC) [home care only]
- Medication Management (MM) [not laboratory]
- National Patient Safety Goals (NPSG)
- Nursing (NR) [critical access hospitals and hospitals only]
- Performance Improvement (PI)
- Provision of Care, Treatment, and Services (PC) [not behavioral health care and human services or laboratory]
- Quality System Assessment for Nonwaived Testing (QSA) [laboratory only]
- Record of Care, Treatment, and Services (RC) [not laboratory]
- Rights and Responsibilities of the Individual (RI) [not laboratory]
- Transplant Safety (TS) [not applicable to assisted living community, behavioral health care and human services, home care, or nursing care centers]
- Waived Testing (WT)

The Joint Commission also has standards manuals for certification and verification programs, all of which are available via E-dition. There are book and/or e-book versions of some of these standards, but not all.

Structure of the Accreditation Requirements

The standard itself is a statement that defines high-level performance expectations, structures, and processes that must be in place for an organization to provide safe, high-quality care, treatment, and services. An organization is scored as either "compliant" or "not compliant" with a standard. Accreditation decisions are based on simple counts of the standards scored "not compliant."

The rationale is a statement that provides background, justification, or additional information about a standard. A standard's rationale is not scored. Not every standard has a written rationale.

Elements of performance (EPs) are specific performance expectations, structures, or processes that must be in place. Every standard has at least one EP. An EP compliance score determines a provider's overall compliance with a standard.

The components of the accreditation requirements are shown in the example on the next page.

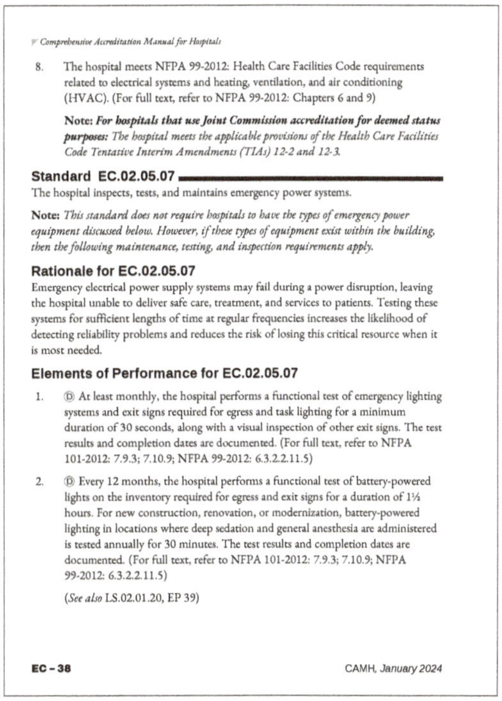

Comprehensive Accreditation Manual for Hospitals

8. The hospital meets NFPA 99-2012: Health Care Facilities Code requirements related to electrical systems and heating, ventilation, and air conditioning (HVAC). (For full text, refer to NFPA 99-2012: Chapters 6 and 9)

   Note: *For hospitals that use Joint Commission accreditation for deemed status purposes:* *The hospital meets the applicable provisions of the Health Care Facilities Code Tentative Interim Amendments (TIAs) 12-2 and 12-3.*

Standard EC.02.05.07

The hospital inspects, tests, and maintains emergency power systems.

Note: *This standard does not require hospitals to have the types of emergency power equipment discussed below. However, if these types of equipment exist within the building, then the following maintenance, testing, and inspection requirements apply.*

Rationale for EC.02.05.07

Emergency electrical power supply systems may fail during a power disruption, leaving the hospital unable to deliver safe care, treatment, and services to patients. Testing these systems for sufficient lengths of time at regular frequencies increases the likelihood of detecting reliability problems and reduces the risk of losing this critical resource when it is most needed.

Elements of Performance for EC.02.05.07

1. Ⓓ At least monthly, the hospital performs a functional test of emergency lighting systems and exit signs required for egress and task lighting for a minimum duration of 30 seconds, along with a visual inspection of other exit signs. The test results and completion dates are documented. (For full text, refer to NFPA 101-2012: 7.9.3; 7.10.9; NFPA 99-2012: 6.3.2.2.11.5)
2. Ⓓ Every 12 months, the hospital performs a functional test of battery-powered lights on the inventory required for egress and exit signs for a duration of 1½ hours. For new construction, renovation, or modernization, battery-powered lighting in locations where deep sedation and general anesthesia are administered is tested annually for 30 minutes. The test results and completion dates are documented. (For full text, refer to NFPA 101-2012: 7.9.3; 7.10.9; NFPA 99-2012: 6.3.2.2.11.5)

   (*See also* LS.02.01.20, EP 39)

EC – 38 CAMH, *January 2024*

Components of a standards chapter in the print manual

E-dition and the Book or E-Book Version of the Manual

The Joint Commission maintains an online version of the standards, known as E-dition, and a book or e-book version of the manual titled the *Comprehensive Accreditation Manual* for a given health care setting. E-dition is complimentary to accredited organizations. Book or e-book versions of the manual are for-sale. Both resources contain the same information. To access the complimentary E-dition, go to Joint Commission Connect. E-dition will be configured and filtered to reflect the standards that apply to your health care organization based on your answers on the e-App. Remember that this version of E-dition is one user at a time, although you can have multiple users from your organization, just not simultaneously. If you need multiple users simultaneously accessing E-dition, you should purchase such access from JCR.

Keeping the Standards Current

Joint Commission standards and EPs generally are updated twice each year for requirements effective January 1 and July 1 of the corresponding year. Revisions are noted in the "What's New" document that appears on E-dition and at the beginning of the book and e-book versions of the *Comprehensive Accreditation Manual*. Additions are also indicated with shading in the *Comprehensive Accreditation Manual* to make changes easier to find, visually, on a page.

These two releases update on E-dition in the fall (for standards effective January 1) and spring (for standards effective July 1), approximately in October and April, respectively. For those that subscribe to the update service for behavioral health care and human services and hospital, replacement pages for the binder version of the *Comprehensive Accreditation Manual* are sent to subscribers.

Occasionally there are interim releases for Joint Commission requirements that must be shared with accredited organizations outside of the normal update cycle. These updates typically address revisions to requirements as they relate to regulatory changes. Interim releases are announced in *Perspectives*. They are available on E-dition and include a "What's New" document of changes as well as the effective date of the requirements.

WHY DO I NEED TO KNOW THIS NOW?

E-dition and the *Comprehensive Accreditation Manual* list all the requirements your organization must comply with. They also provide support resources, such as the ACC chapter, that you can reference at any time.

WHERE DO I START?

- **Get to know the standards.** Visit E-dition or read through your *Comprehensive Accreditation Manual*. Familiarize yourself with how this content is presented and what content is provided.
- **Read Joint Commission *Perspectives*.** This newsletter is published monthly and provides information about revisions and updates to Joint Commission standards, policies, and other requirements. *Perspectives* is considered official, legal communication of all updated, revised, and/or new requirements; therefore, accredited organizations should read it monthly to ensure that they are aware of any changes to requirements, policies, or procedures. All Joint Commission-accredited, -certified, and -verified organizations receive complimentary access via their secure *Joint Commission Connect* extranet site and may share the newsletter within the organization.

KEY CONCEPT

SURVEY READINESS

The survey process is a comprehensive evaluation of all aspects of an organization's function. It requires the participation of many staff members and the delivery of a great deal of information. You will want to prepare for your survey to ensure that it goes as smoothly as possible, with minimal disruption to normal operations and as little extra work for busy staff members as possible.

Survey Readiness Committee

One way you can ensure that your organization is properly prepared for its next survey is to form a Survey Readiness Committee. It is not required that you do this. For some organizations it will suffice to have an accreditation professional or two, or a small team, perform the functions of a Survey Readiness Committee. But for larger or more complex organizations, it is recommended that a cross-disciplinary committee be formed to prepare for the survey and assemble information for the surveyors.

PICTURE THIS

Identifying Standards Applicability

Standard/ Requirement Number	EP #	Ambulatory Surgery Centers	Endoscopy	Medical Centers	Dental Centers	Diagnostic/Therapeutic	Diagnostic Imaging Services	Diagnostic Sleep Centers	Kidney Care/Dialysis	Telehealth/Nonsurgical	Telehealth/Surgical	Episodic Care	Occupational/Worksite Health	Urgent/Immediate Care	Convenient Care
	4	X	X	X	X	X	X	X	X	X	X	X	X	X	X
	5	X	X	X	X	X	X	X	X	X	X	X	X	X	X
	6	X	X												
LD.04.02.03	1	X	X	X	X	X	X	X	X	X	X	X	X	X	X
	5	X	X	X	X	X	X	X	X	X	X	X	X	X	X
	7	X	X	X	X	X	X	X	X	X	X	X	X	X	X
	10	X	X	X	X	X	X	X		X	X	X	X	X	X
LD.04.03.01	1	X	X	X	X	X	X	X	X	X	X	X	X	X	X
	25	X	X												
LD.04.03.09	1	X	X	X	X	X	X	X	X	X	X	X	X	X	X
	2	X	X	X	X	X	X	X	X	X	X	X	X	X	X
	3	X	X	X	X	X	X	X	X	X	X	X	X	X	X
	4	X	X	X	X	X	X	X	X	X	X	X	X	X	X
	5	X	X	X	X	X	X	X	X	X	X	X	X	X	X
	6	X	X	X	X	X	X	X	X	X	X	X	X	X	X
	7	X	X	X	X	X	X	X	X	X	X	X	X	X	X
	8	X	X	X	X	X	X	X	X	X	X	X	X	X	X
	10	X	X	X	X	X	X	X	X	X	X	X	X	X	X
LD.04.03.13	1	X		X	X				X			X		X	
	3	X		X	X				X			X		X	
	4	X		X	X				X			X		X	
	6			X	X				X			X		X	
LS.01.01.01	1	X	X		X										
	2	X	X												
	3	X	X												
	4	X	X												
	6	X	X												
	7	X	X												
LS.01.02.01	1	X	X												
	2	X	X												
	3	X	X												
	4	X	X												
	5	X	X												
	6	X	X												
	7	X	X												
	8	X	X												

Note that not all standards apply to all organizations covered under the manual. Depending on the services your organization provides, some standards may apply, and others may not. A Standards Applicability Grid (Process), like the one shown here, is included in most *Comprehensive Accreditation Manuals* to clarify what standards are applicable within a specific health care setting. The grid is your guide to which standards apply to your organization and which do not.

If you use E-dition, the standards not applicable to your organization, based on information provided in your E-App, will be hidden from view automatically. You also can apply a filter in E-dition to further screen the standards you see.

Here is one approach to that kind of committee:

- **Membership.** Identify (or call for nominations of) a chair and cochair to coordinate the committee. The organization's accreditation lead should be one of those, but not necessarily the chair. The chair should have the support of all levels of leadership. Solicit remaining committee members from appointed clinical experts, managers, and directors identified by your leaders. As a committee, you can determine how to make sure every manual chapter's requirements are considered. Rotate membership as needed.
- **Attendance.** Make sure every committee member understands the need to commit to attending meetings or sending substitutes if necessary. Replace frequently absent or inactive members promptly.
- **Clear and simple goals.** As a committee, establish a scope of responsibility to the organization and committee goals. Keep goals to a minimum to cover core functions/activities. And make them clear and simple: They're easier to keep in mind and share/promote.
- **Responsibilities.**
    - **Chairs.** The chairs should meet with the executive-level leaders to give standards compliance reports (likely at board meetings; sometimes quarterly, sometimes every six months, depending on the survey period). The chairs may also meet before and after with senior leaders to share information and ideas for compliance.
    - **Other members.** Members will be more committed if they have clearly defined responsibilities—reporting data, sharing information from the field, and so on. Who, besides the chairs or chapter leaders (staff members who have been given the responsibility to oversee compliance with the requirements in a specific accreditation standards chapter), for example, will evaluate compliance? What data—and from whom—does the committee need to support the evaluation?
- **Frequency.** It's a good idea for the committee to meet every few weeks at first. Then, when everyone is clear about expectations, you can meet bimonthly or quarterly, depending on your survey cycle. You may also want to meet after significant performance improvement (PI) projects to share results for discussion and make recommendations for further actions, including reporting to leaders.
- **Reports.** You may have a variety of reports from PI teams and tracer teams (see "Mock Tracer Program" below) to review at each meeting. The information should clearly relate not only to specific Joint Commission standards but also to committee goals and objectives.
- **Results.** Both positive and negative compliance results from Joint Commission surveys and internal reports should be shared outside the committee. But protocol is important: Leaders may wish to hear reports first. With guidance from leaders, share compliance results with the rest of the organization.

Mock Tracer Program

Another way to maintain survey readiness is to operate a mock tracer program within your organization. Tracers are tools surveyors use to evaluate overall operations; they take an in-depth look at actual organization functions. They can focus on a specific process, such as medical device sterilization, or they can follow an individual receiving care through their course of care, treatment, and services. It all depends on what you want to assess. You can run mock tracers to evaluate your own operations and help guide PI and compliance activities. Each year in *Perspectives* The Joint Commission publishes the top 10 Requirements for Improvement (RFIs) by program. This list can be a great starting point for mock tracers. (For more on tracer methodology, see page 49.)

Whatever you choose to focus your tracers on, make sure the process includes the following critical steps:

- **Identify deficiencies.** Either by talking with staff or through the tracer process itself, collect deficiency data to show patterns and trends and identify areas or processes that require improvement.
- **Develop corrective actions.** Work with knowledgeable staff to identify changes that will improve performance.
- **Assign staff to carry out corrective actions.** To make sure intended changes are implemented, you should explicitly identify who does what.
- **Set dates for accountability.** Make sure that everyone involved knows when they are expected to have implemented changes, when the efficacy of changes will be assessed, and when the process may be reevaluated.

TOOL

Comprehensive Organization Assessment Tool

Using software, such as Tracers with AMP®, is an efficient way to conduct mock tracers and aggregate and analyze the data to identify areas for improvement. Please note that Tracers with AMP is a for-sale product from JCR and its use is not required for Joint Commission accreditation. It is mentioned here primarily for your information only.

For more information on tracers, *see* "Tracer Methodology" in Chapter 4.

Survey Activity Guide

A critical resource for survey readiness is the *Survey Activity Guide*. This guide is published annually by The Joint Commission and posted on its website (and on organizations' *Joint Commission Connect* extranet sites). At times there are midyear updates; these are posted on organizations' *Joint Commission Connect* extranet sites. The *Survey Activity Guide* breaks down the survey process into its constituent parts, lets you know what all the survey activities are, what order you can expect them to happen in, and what materials or support will be required for each. Note that the *Survey Activity Guide*s are program specific. If your organization has more than one accredited program, you will need to download all applicable *Survey Activity Guide*s.

Survey Practice

Practice makes perfect, or at least better. One good way to get ready for and reduce anxiety of a survey is to practice the process in your own organization. That way, when the surveyors arrive, you and the staff will know better what to expect. Here are some important elements to include in your survey practice:

- **Tour the environment.** This is not required by The Joint Commission, but referencing the *Survey Activity Guide*, you can get a sense of where the surveyors will want to go and what they will want to see. Try planning and conducting mock surveys to identify compliance issues and accustom staff to being observed and questioned about their activities and responsibilities.

Mock tracers and real tracers are looking to see what staff know—not to "catch" them in an error.

- **Identify who participates in which sessions.** Just as in any other area of the organization's operations, everyone needs to be clear as to what their role is in the survey process and their specific responsibilities.
- **Schedule tours, mock tracers, and any other survey-related items as identified.** Rely on the *Survey Activity Guide* to plan and schedule survey-related activities. Even if you don't do a full mock survey, knowing how everyone is going to make time for survey activities is an important part of readiness.
- **Plan initial meeting with surveyors.** Who will greet the surveyors? Who will be notified immediately of their arrival? Who will escort them to their work space? These and other questions about the surveyors' initial arrival at the facility should be answered ahead of time, rather than on an ad hoc basis during a real survey. Practice the process from the moment surveyors show up at your front door. This would involve reception, admitting, security, and other staff. Practice assembling the initial survey documents as outlined in the *Survey Activity Guide*. In some cases, the surveyor may ask for documentation that you do not have readily available. The surveyor will allow you to use an IOU, but the surveyor will stipulate when the IOU is due to them. Practice how to manage IOUs so you are sure to provide the missing documentation within the listed time frame.
- **Prepare staff.** Let staff know what to expect when the surveyors come around. Share parts of this book and emphasize the collaborative nature of the survey process. This is not an interrogation or an attempt to find fault with their performance. It is a performance improvement and quality assessment exercise in which they have a key role to play. Encourage honesty and transparency. This is staff's opportunity to shine and show off what they know. Encourage positivity, not fear.

Required Documents

Due to the nature of the survey process and the fact that many of the standards require documentation of processes or activities, surveyors will require a great deal of documents and information at the time of the survey. As previously noted, you should review the standards on E-dition or in your *Comprehensive Accreditation Manual*, with special attention to those requirements that specifically require documentation. These are marked with a Ⓓ icon and are also listed in the "Required Written Documentation" (RWD) chapter in your *Comprehensive Accreditation Manual*, if applicable. If you are working with E-dition, you can filter the standards so that you see only those that require documentation. Also, the *Survey Activity Guide* contains a wealth of information that will help you prepare the information and documentation surveyors will need and when. Another good resource is *PolicySource*™, which features dozens of downloadable, sample policies and procedures reviewed and approved by The Joint Commission. *PolicySource* is a for-sale resource from JCR; it is mentioned here for your information only. Its use is not required by The Joint Commission.

TOOL

Checklist for Evaluating Policy and Procedure Templates

Postponing a Survey

For initial surveys, your organization may contact your account executive to change the "ready" date submitted in the application at any time prior to the scheduling of the initial survey. After the survey is scheduled, you have 20 business days to request a postponement without financial penalty. After 20 business days, a penalty is incurred if you request the postponement of a scheduled initial survey. For resurveys, an organization can postpone the survey without financial penalty only in the event of a major disruption, such as a natural disaster, a major employee strike, or moving the organization or program to a new location. If none of these criteria are met and your organization still wishes to postpone its survey, at the discretion of The Joint Commission, the survey may be postponed for a fee so long as it is more than 20 days before the first day of the scheduled survey.

WHY DO I NEED TO KNOW THIS NOW?

If you demonstrate leadership in survey readiness now and the result is a good survey, you're likely to get more support for the next survey. And even if your first survey has a few bumps, you'll earn the trust and respect of leaders and staff by showing you know the importance of being prepared.

TOOL

Daily Compliance Checklist

WHERE DO I START?

- **Learn more.** Take time to review The Joint Commission's *Survey Activity Guide*. It's focused to get you prepared for what happens during a survey. Ask your account executive if you have any questions about what you learn.
- **Facilitate processes.** Use a checklist designed to prepare for a surveyor's visit to practice the procedures.
- **Check documentation.** Use E-dition to do a filtered search for the Ⓓ icon or review the "Required Written Documentation" (RWD) chapter in your *Comprehensive Accreditation Manual* (if applicable) to determine what documentation is required. Be sure the required written documentation is on hand if a surveyor asks to see it.
- **Get organized.** If your organization doesn't already have an accreditation committee or compliance review project team, you might want to form one. Remember to work with your peers, ask for help from your mentor or supervisor, and be mindful of organization politics. Above all, work to get leaders on board from the start.

Test Your Knowledge

1. Which is your official source of communication with The Joint Commission about your organization's accreditation?
   - ☐ a. E-dition®
   - ☐ b. *Joint Commission Connect®*
   - ☐ c. *Survey Activity Guide*
   - ☐ d. *Comprehensive Accreditation Manual*
2. Which of the following is your primary resource for Joint Commission accreditation standards and other requirements?
   - ☐ a. E-dition
   - ☐ b. *Joint Commission Connect*
   - ☐ c. *Survey Activity Guide*
   - ☐ d. Joint Commission account executive
3. Which of the following is your primary resource for determining whether a component or service of your health care organization needs to be included with your accreditation application?
   - ☐ a. E-dition
   - ☐ b. *Joint Commission Connect*
   - ☐ c. *Survey Activity Guide*
   - ☐ d. Your Joint Commission account executive
4. Which of the following is your primary resource for an outline of topics and activities during a survey?
   - ☐ a. E-dition
   - ☐ b. *Joint Commission Connect*
   - ☐ c. *Survey Activity Guide*
   - ☐ d. Your Joint Commission account executive
5. How quickly must you update The Joint Commission of any significant changes to your organization?
   - ☐ a. Within 7 days
   - ☐ b. Within 15 days
   - ☐ c. Within 30 days
   - ☐ d. When an additional service is contemplated
6. Which of the following entities requires you to request "deemed status" if you are using The Joint Commission to meet their program requirements? (Select all that apply.)
   - ☐ a. Centers for Medicare & Medicaid Services
   - ☐ b. Substance Abuse and Mental Health Services Administration
   - ☐ c. American College of Surgeons' trauma certification
   - ☐ d. Health plan participation

(continued)

7. What does CCN stand for?
   - ☐ a. Condition of Certification Number
   - ☐ b. Continuous Compliance Nomenclature
   - ☐ c. CMS Certification Number
8. Generally, how often are Joint Commission standards updated?
   - ☐ a. Once a year
   - ☐ b. Twice a year
   - ☐ c. Quarterly
   - ☐ d. Monthly
9. What does the D icon in Joint Commission standards indicate?
   - ☐ a. Demonstration required
   - ☐ b. Diagnosis required
   - ☐ c. Documentation required

The Survey

CHAPTER 4

THE BIG IDEA

The Joint Commission offers a variety of tools to help health care organizations monitor their own compliance with standards and improve performance, but the survey is the in-depth evaluation of the organization's performance in meeting the standards for accreditation. Once every three years (two years for laboratories) Joint Commission surveyors will show up at your door unannounced, and you will be required to provide them with information and data about your operations, and access to your care recipients, staff, and facilities or wherever care, treatment, or services are provided. This chapter should give you an idea of what to expect during the survey process.

KEY CONCEPTS

- What You Can Expect
- Tracer Methodology

THE MANUAL

Following are the relevant Joint Commission E-dition® or *Comprehensive Accreditation Manual* chapters:

- "Accreditation Participation Requirements" (APR)
- "The Accreditation Process" (ACC)

KEY CONCEPT

WHAT YOU CAN EXPECT

Observe processes, review documents, ask questions, take notes, offer strategies, provide feedback, and create reports. That's what accreditation professionals do daily to serve care recipients. And that's pretty much what Joint Commission surveyors do during a survey.

"I heard that...
new organizations need to be surveyed immediately."

fact:
The key issue is when you feel you will be ready for your survey. A new organization will need to be surveyed within 12 months of submitting its application and deposit. We will do our best to schedule your survey on or after the month you indicate on the application as your "ready date." Most organizations request to be surveyed 3–9 months after they have submitted their application to give themselves time to prepare. But we can also be responsive to short turnaround times for those who wish to be surveyed more quickly.

Types of Surveys

Just what will your survey be like? Well, that depends on your organization, which accreditation program it will be surveyed under, and other factors. The following list summarizes the various types of surveys conducted. You may experience several different types of surveys. (See the ACC chapter of E-dition or the *Comprehensive Accreditation Manual* for further elaboration on each type of survey and related policies.)

- **Initial survey.** This is for fully functioning organizations that haven't sought accreditation before and are ready for a full survey or for those that are seeking deemed status.
- **Reaccreditation survey.** After your organization receives its initial accreditation, you will be subject to reaccreditation surveys at least every 36 months (24 months for laboratories).
- **Additional survey types.**
  - **Extension survey.** This is conducted when an accredited organization adds a new service, program, or site that significantly changes how it delivers care or expands its scope of care. The goal is to make sure the previous accreditation status is still appropriate.
  - **For-cause survey.** This is done when The Joint Commission becomes aware of a potentially serious compliance, care, or safety issue.
  - **Follow-up survey for a condition-level deficiency.** This occurs based on condition-level deficiency findings only.

TOOL

Procedure Checklist for First-Day-of-Survey Readiness

Survey Agenda

The Joint Commission provides a sample survey agenda for your organization posted on your organization's *Joint Commission Connect®* extranet site. The agenda lists all the major sessions and activities that are to take place during your survey. After you have completed and submitted your electronic application for accreditation (E-App) and The Joint Commission processes it, you will have a better idea of what the survey agenda might be for your organization. You may request minor alterations to the agenda when the surveyors arrive, but the broad outlines are fixed. The *Survey Activity Guide* has Survey Activity Lists for each setting or program that can help you know what kinds of activities to expect and plan to make the appropriate staff available for scheduled survey activities. The *Survey Activity Guide* also contains requested documentation lists for each health care setting so that you can plan to have the proper documentation ready when the surveyors request it. In some instances, you may be asked to upload certain documents to a secure portal for surveyors to review before they arrive at your organization. However, this is not yet widespread practice for all accreditation programs. Your account representative will be able to guide you, as will your program's *Survey Activity Guide*.

Meet the Team

Each survey will begin with the arrival of one or more surveyors at your site. Staff at the front desk should know what to do when this happens. We have included a short tool in this chapter to remind those frontline staff what the correct procedure is when Joint Commission surveyors show up. Briefly, they need to greet the surveyors and verify their identities by requesting Joint Commission photo identification. They should then ask the surveyors to wait in a preselected location while the relevant staff are located and notified. At this point the most important people to contact are the person with the *Joint Commission Connect* password, who can log in to the system and verify that the survey event is scheduled, and the staff member designated to escort the survey team to its workspace.

"I heard that...

if my organization disagrees with a Joint Commission surveyor during a survey, my organization automatically loses the disagreement."

fact

If your organization and a Joint Commission surveyor are in disagreement on an issue, you can request that you call the Joint Commission Standards Interpretation Group together.

PICTURE THIS

Hospital Accreditation – Sample Agenda

Session/Activity Name	Expected Duration of Activity
Surveyor Arrival and Preliminary Planning (includes the Safety Briefing)	30–60 minutes
Opening Conference	15 minutes
Orientation to Organization	30–60 minutes
Individual Tracers	60–120 minutes
Program-Specific Tracers	60–120 minutes
System Tracers	30–90 minutes
Issue Resolution or Surveyor Planning/Team Meeting	30 minutes
Daily Briefing	15–60 minutes
Emergency Management Session	45–90 minutes
Leadership Session	60 minutes
Competence Assessment and Credentialing and Privileging	60–120 minutes
Report Preparation	60–120 minutes
Exit Briefing	15 minutes
Exit Conference	30 minutes

These activities are the building blocks of your survey agenda. Review the *Survey Activity Guide* for more information, including program-specific activities.

Nursing Care Center Accreditation – Sample Agenda

DAY 1

Time	Activity
8:00 – 8:30 a.m.	Surveyor Arrival and Preliminary Planning Session
8:30 – 9:00 a.m.	• Opening Conference and Orientation to Organization • Brief Orientation Tour of the Organization
9:00 – 9:30 a.m.	
9:30 – 10:00 a.m.	Individual Tracer Activity
10:00 – 10:30 a.m.	
10:30 – 11:00 a.m.	
11:00 – 11:30 a.m.	
11:30 – 12:00 p.m.	
12:00 – 12:30 p.m.	Surveyor Lunch
12:30 – 1:00 p.m.	Individual Tracer Activity
1:00 – 1:30 p.m.	
1:30 – 2:00 p.m.	
2:00 – 2:30 p.m.	
2:30 – 3:00 p.m.	Environment of Care and Emergency Management
3:00 – 3:30 p.m.	
3:30 – 4:00 p.m.	Life Safety Building Tour (Abbreviated)
4:00 – 4:30 p.m.	Special Issue Resolution OR Surveyor Planning/Team Meeting

DAY 2

Time	Activity
8:00 – 8:30 a.m.	Daily Briefing
8:30 – 9:00 a.m.	Leadership and Data Use Session This session will focus on: • Leadership's role and use of data in maintaining systems, infrastructure, and key processes that contribute to the quality and safety of resident and patient care • Leadership's use of data and related activities for evaluating and improving the organization's culture of providing person-centered care • The organization's performance improvement process • The use of data in providing safe and quality care such as the following: - Infection control - Medication management - MDS performance - Resident and staff perceptions on the provision of person-centered care
9:00 – 9:30 a.m.	
9:30 – 10:00 a.m.	
10:00 – 10:30 a.m.	Individual Tracer Activity
10:30 – 11:00 a.m.	
11:00 – 11:30 a.m.	
11:30 – 12:00 p.m.	Competence Assessment Session
12:00 – 12:30 p.m.	Credentialing of Physicians and Other Licensed Practitioners
12:30 – 1:00 p.m.	Surveyor Lunch
1:00 – 1:30 p.m.	Individual Tracer Activity
1:30 – 2:00 p.m.	
2:00 – 2:30 p.m.	
2:30 – 3:00 p.m.	
3:00 – 3:30 p.m.	Surveyor Report Preparation
3:30 – 4:00 p.m.	
4:00 – 4:30 p.m.	CEO Exit Briefing and Organization Exit Conference

Survey Length

The length of a survey is anywhere from one to five days. The length of the survey varies according to the size and complexity of your organization. For example, *Life Safety Code*®* survey lengths are determined by your organization's square footage, including support areas such as lab, kitchen, mechanical spaces, pharmacy, and laundry. A survey with a more limited scope that is not your reaccreditation survey may take as little as one day.

WHY DO I NEED TO KNOW THIS NOW?

The survey process is a rigorous look at your organization's standards compliance. It requires you to provide a great deal of access and documentation in a relatively short amount of time. Being familiar with the process before it starts and having a plan for managing the survey will make the process go a lot more smoothly for everyone.

WHERE DO I START?

- ***Learn more.*** Familiarize yourself with the *Survey Activity Guide*. If you have never worked on a survey before, it is the best way to learn what to expect and what will be expected of you.
- **Work with your team.** Reach out regularly to the members of your Survey Readiness Committee, if you have one, or anyone you will be relying on to help with the survey process, such as chapter leaders. Make sure required documentation is up to date and that everyone is aware of any possible compliance issues.
- **Keep staff in the loop.** The more information about the process and what is required of them, the better able they will be to provide useful information and work with surveyors with a minimum of stress and disruption.

"I heard that...

all Joint Commission surveys are unannounced."

fact

Although all deemed status surveys are unannounced, there are instances in which survey dates or ranges will be known. Your initial survey will be scheduled in collaboration with The Joint Commission according to your "ready date." Also, surveys conducted as part of the Early Survey Policy will be announced surveys. Non-deemed programs may receive a seven-day advance notice of a survey.

EXCEPTIONS TO UNANNOUNCED SURVEYS

The following bullets list the exceptions to unannounced Joint Commission surveys. Note that exceptions do not apply if your organization is tailored with another program that is not eligible for an announced survey or if an unannounced survey is required for deemed status purposes.

Announced Surveys

- First survey conducted by The Joint Commission
- First survey conducted under the Early Survey Policy
- Focused Standards Assessment Options 2 and 3 surveys

Organizations That Receive Seven-Day Notice of Surveys

- Ambulatory Care
    - Office-based surgery practices
    - Telehealth services
    - Sleep centers
    - Ambulatory surgery centers not using accreditation for deemed status
    - Ambulatory care organizations providing only one of the following services:

* *Life Safety Code*® is a registered trademark of the National Fire Protection Association, Quincy, MA.

    - Surgery/anesthesia services
    - Medical/dental services with fewer than 5,000 annual visits or fewer than three licensed practitioners
    - Specified diagnostic/therapeutic services* with fewer than 3,000 annual visits or four or fewer licensed practitioners
    - Mobile diagnostic services
- Behavioral Health Care and Human Services
  - Correction settings
  - Child welfare programs
  - Methadone programs
  - Behavioral health care and human services organizations with fewer than 10 staff or an average daily census fewer than 100:
    - "Small" settings
    - Outpatient and day programs
    - 24-hour services
    - In-home behavioral health, case management, or assertive community treatment program
    - Inpatient, freestanding organizations
    - Community-based, freestanding organizations
    - Inpatient crisis stabilization programs
    - Residential/group homes

- Home Care
  - Home care organizations with only one of the following services*:
    - Home health/personal care/support services
    - Hospice
    - Pharmacy
    - Home medical equipment services (except when using accreditation to meet Medicare DMEPOS† requirements)
    - Home infusion therapy

- Laboratory
  - "Small" organizations with fewer than 25,000 tests per year
  - Freestanding in vitro fertilization laboratories

- Other Facilities
  - US Department of Defense facilities
  - US Bureau of Prisons facilities
  - Immigration facilities

* This includes allergy, alternative/complementary care, audiology, chiropractic medicine, diagnostic imaging, dialysis, hematology, infusion therapy, lithotripsy, orthotics/prosthetics, pain management, physical medicine, pulmonary medicine, and radiation oncology.

† DMEPOS, durable medical equipment, prosthetics, orthotics, and supplies.

KEY CONCEPT

TRACER METHODOLOGY

By tracking or tracing the path of a care recipient through their course of treatment, across the continuum of care, or if by tracing a critical organization process from its beginning to its end, surveyors and accreditation professionals can gain valuable information about how well the organization is complying with standards.

What Are Tracers?

Tracers are the primary tool used by surveyors for surveys. Tracers are basically a way for Joint Commission surveyors, or the organization's own accreditation professionals in the case of mock tracers, to audit operations in a way that is at once specific and holistic. Each type is defined below. Which types of tracers surveyors choose to use depends on what kind of organization is being surveyed and what the surveyors observe. You'll find that one tracer can lead to another.

What Is Expected of Staff During Tracers?

During an individual tracer, the surveyor will review the care recipient's electronic health record (EHR);* observe the delivery of care, treatment, and services provided to the individual; and interview staff about their duties and their care and treatment of the individual. Staff are expected to provide clear and honest answers to surveyor questions; deliver care, treatment, and services as they normally would, in compliance with Joint Commission standards; and work with the surveyor to protect the rights and privacy of those receiving care, treatment, and services during the survey process. Each surveyor should be assigned an escort to help them navigate the facility. And one or more information technology (IT) or data science professionals should provide documents and data to the survey team and solve any IT problems that may arise.

Types of Tracers

There are three types of tracers:

- **Individual tracer.** In this type of tracer, a surveyor tracks the care, treatment, and services a specific care recipient has received at your organization. This type of tracer is used to analyze (1) how individual components of your systems provide care for individuals, and (2) how those systems interact with each other. It's the most common type of tracer. Note: Something a surveyor observes during an individual tracer can prompt the need for a system tracer or an environment of care tracer. Laboratory programs use only individual tracers.
- **System tracer.** In this type of tracer, a surveyor analyzes one specific high-risk system or process across your entire organization. These tracers focus on care recipients' care, treatment, and services whenever possible.

* The Joint Commission does not require health records to be electronic.

Unlike the individual tracer, which follows a care recipient moving among systems, a system tracer evaluates the system itself as it relates to individuals receiving care. System tracers may address infection prevention and control, data management, and/or medication management. Although the environment of care tracer isn't a defined system tracer, it is similar and focuses on the physical environment of a health care organization.

- **Program-specific tracer.** In this type of tracer, a surveyor focuses on topics pertinent to a specific program or service your organization provides, examining the different levels and types of care and identifying safety concerns. See the next page for a list of some program-specific tracers.

WHY DO I NEED TO KNOW THIS NOW?

Tracers are a critical component to surveys that lead surveyors to determine if an organization is complying with Joint Commission standards.

WHERE DO I START?

- **Talk with staff.** If you are new to accreditation, reach out to staff members who have been a part of a previous Joint Commission survey. These individuals may be a valuable resource as you acclimate to your new position.
- **Review past notes and survey reports.** If your organization is already accredited or certified by The Joint Commission, look through any notes from past accreditation professionals; your predecessor may have conducted mock tracers that you can implement. You may also review past survey reports, if available, to see what was observed.
- **Use software.** Tracers with AMP® enables you to access user-friendly, interactive dashboards and easy-to-build automated reports to help you proactively identify risk areas, prioritize improvements, compare key performance indicators, document changes, and track progress over time. Hospitals, critical access hospitals, and ambulatory surgery centers can add the Centers for Medicare & Medicaid (CMS) module to manage both Joint Commission accreditation and CMS compliance with one tool. Please note that Tracers with AMP is a for-sale product from JCR, and its use is not required for Joint Commission accreditation. It is mentioned here for your information only.

PICTURE THIS

Types of Program-Specific Tracers

Continuity of Care (AC)
Elopement (BHC)
Continuity of Foster/Therapeutic Foster Care (BHC)
Violence (BHC)
Suicide Prevention (BHC; HAP)
Laboratory Integration (CAH; HAP)
Patient Flow (CAH; HAP)
Staffing (NCC)
Equipment and Supply Management (OME)
Fall Reduction (OME)
Hospital Readmission (OME)

These are examples of program-specific tracers that may be conducted during your organization's survey. These tracers may be included on your survey agenda or they may be added because of a surveyor observation. The program-specific tracers are subject to change. Refer to your *Survey Activity Guide*.

AC, Ambulatory Care; BHC, Behavioral Health Care and Human Services; CAH, Critical Access Hospitals; HAP, Hospitals; NCC, Nursing Care Centers; OME, Home Care.

Test Your Knowledge

1. Which of the following tells you how many surveyors could be involved in your organization's survey?
   - ☐ a. E-dition®
   - ☐ b. *Survey Activity Guide*
   - ☐ c. E-App
   - ☐ d. Survey agenda
2. What is The Joint Commission's technique for evaluating compliance during survey?
   - ☐ a. Tracer methodology
   - ☐ b. Socratic inquiry
   - ☐ c. Learning checks
   - ☐ d. Random, periodic interviews
3. Which of the following is the type of survey you would request if you added a new clinical site or divested part of your home care program from a current existing accredited organization?
   - ☐ a. For cause
   - ☐ b. Validation
   - ☐ c. Extension
   - ☐ d. Triennial
4. All Joint Commission surveys are unannounced.
   - ☐ a. True
   - ☐ b. False

After a Joint Commission Survey

CHAPTER 5

THE BIG IDEA

So you made it through the survey. Now what? Well, two weeks to two months after the survey you can expect an accreditation decision from The Joint Commission. This chapter will give you an overview of how those decisions are made and what kinds of corrective actions The Joint Commission may require of your organization.

KEY CONCEPTS

- The Scoring Process
- Follow-Up Activities
- Accreditation Outcomes

THE MANUAL

Following is the relevant Joint Commission E-dition® or *Comprehensive Accreditation Manual* chapter:

- "The Accreditation Process" (ACC)

KEY CONCEPT

THE SCORING PROCESS

Accreditation decisions will be made according to the level of compliance with Joint Commission standards observed by the surveyors. Where the surveyors find the organization out of compliance with the standards, they will evaluate the scope and assess the risk posed by the noncompliance and convey that information in the accreditation report.

PICTURE THIS

Survey Analysis for Evaluating Risk® (*SAFER®*) Matrix

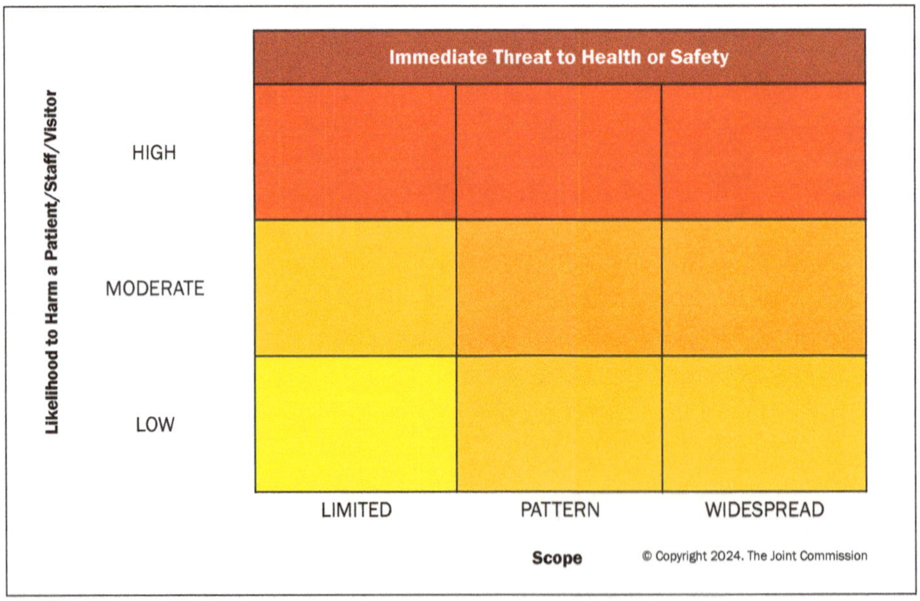

The *SAFER* Matrix was developed to help organizations assess the risk posed by noncompliance with standards cited on survey. Any noncompliant standards from your survey will be posted on a *SAFER* Matrix. You can also use this matrix as a tool to evaluate what compliance issues your organization has and where to focus performance improvement activities. The following table provides definitions for the likelihood to harm and scope categories.

Category	Definition	Further Guidance
Scope		
Limited	Unique occurrence that is not representative of routine/regular practice and has the potential to affect only one or a very limited number of patients, visitors, or staff.	An Outlier • Scope is isolated when one or a very limited number of patients are affected and/or one or a very limited number of staff are involved and/or the deficiency occurs in a very limited number of locations.
Pattern	Multiple occurrences of the deficiency or a single occurrence that has the potential to affect more than a limited number of patients, visitors, or staff.	Process Variation • Scope is pattern when more than a very limited number of patients are affected, more than a very limited number of staff are involved, the situation has occurred in several locations, and/or the same patient(s) has been affected by repeated occurrences of the same deficient practice.
Widespread	Deficiency is pervasive in the facility, represents systemic failure, or has the potential to affect most/all patients, visitors, or staff.	Process Failure • Scope is widespread when the deficiency affects most/all patients, is pervasive in the facility, or represents systemic failure. Widespread scope refers to the entire organization, not just a subset of patients or one unit.
Likelihood to Harm		
Low	Harm could happen but would be rare.	• Undermines safety/quality or contributes to an unsafe environment but very unlikely to directly contribute to harm. • It would be rare for any actual patient harm to occur as a result of the deficiency.
Moderate	Harm could happen occasionally.	• Could cause harm directly but more likely to cause harm as a contributing factor in the presence of special circumstances or additional failures. • If the deficiency continues, it would be possible that harm could occur, but only in certain situations and/or patients.
High	Harm could happen at any time.	• Could directly lead to harm without the need for other significant circumstances or failures. • If the deficiency continues, it would be likely that harm could happen at any time to any patient (or did actually happen).

The *SAFER* Matrix

There are many standards to comply with to achieve and maintain Joint Commission accreditation. Some of them can be rather challenging. Finding out you are noncompliant with a standard presents an opportunity to come into compliance. You will usually be given time to bring the organization into compliance. To help you prioritize which findings to address first, The Joint Commission developed the *Survey Analysis for Evaluating Risk® (SAFER®)* Matrix. The surveyor who finds evidence of noncompliance will rate the noncompliance by using this matrix according to the likelihood that it will cause harm and how wide the scope of the problem may be. Each noncompliant standard will be assigned a value on the vertical axis corresponding to low, moderate, or high likelihood to cause harm, and each will be assigned a value on the horizontal axis corresponding to the scope of the issue being limited, pattern, or widespread. As you move from the lower left corner to the upper right corner, standards cited represent higher risk. Those are the Requirements for Improvement (RFIs) that demand your attention and should be prioritized in performance improvement activities.

TOOL

Survey Analysis for Evaluating Risk® (SAFER®) Matrix

SAFER Dashboard

A *SAFER* Matrix–related Joint Commission platform—the *SAFER* Dashboard—empowers users to look at their survey performance data through multiple lenses. This data analytics tool is available free to accredited organizations via their *Joint Commission Connect*® extranet site.

The synergy of multiple perspectives, from macro to micro, in data analysis can help an organization determine the most effective and efficient corrective measures and long-term action plans for performance improvement. Uncovering previously unseen patterns enables organizations to implement targeted, customized solutions.

Accreditation Reports

In addition to the *SAFER* Matrix, the accreditation report will contain detailed information about each finding of noncompliance. This will include a description of how the organization is noncompliant with the standard in question, sometimes called the surveyor's findings or observations. For more information on corrective action, *see* "Follow-Up Activities" on page 57.

How Accreditation Decisions Are Made

Accreditation decisions are made based on standards compliance, as observed during the survey, and the presence of any repeat findings from previous survey activity, along with any patterns, trends, or themes.

WHY DO I NEED TO KNOW THIS NOW?

The survey is a collaborative evaluation of performance and standards compliance. The *SAFER* Matrix and the accreditation report are your guides to addressing areas where your organization needs to improve.

WHERE DO I START?

- **Gather documents.** Use the accreditation report information and the underlying data and documentation you supplied to the surveyors to gain better understanding of why the organization is not in compliance.
- **Talk to surveyors.** During the survey, use the surveyors as the expert resources they are. They bring a wealth of experience and expertise in the industry. They are there to help.
- **Seek expert help.** Sometimes it will be hard to understand how to apply a certain standard in the context of your organization. Where you find the standards hard to interpret, check out The Joint Commission's Standards Interpretation Group Frequently Asked Questions (FAQs) online. This group provides guidance on the interpretation and application of the standards to health care organizations and Joint Commission staff.

"I heard that...

accreditation is either granted or denied based on the survey."

fact

Yes, although your surveyor does not render a decision at the time of survey. A final accreditation decision, based primarily on survey findings, will not be rendered until all required follow-up activity has been completed. The team making the decision also will consider follow-up activities and Joint Commission staff recommendations. Accreditation and Denial of Accreditation are only two of the possible decisions that may be rendered following survey. It is also possible that your organization will receive Accreditation with Follow-up Survey or Preliminary Denial of Accreditation. Compliance is an ongoing project. Each of these accreditation decisions carries with it specific requirements and next steps toward accreditation. Even a grant of accreditation may carry with it a Requirement for Improvement (RFI) and perhaps required Evidence of Standards Compliance (ESC). *See* "Follow-Up Activities" on page 57 for more information. *See* page 59 for an example of a completed ESC. *See* "Accreditation Outcomes" on page 61 for more information about different types of accreditation decisions.

KEY CONCEPT

FOLLOW-UP ACTIVITIES

Joint Commission surveys are intended to be a partnership between the organization and surveyors, with the primary objective being to find any potential risk to care recipients based on processes observed. So chances are you are going to have some work to do following your survey to address specific areas of improvement identified in your accreditation survey report.

Requirements for Improvement

Shortly after your survey is completed, an accreditation report will be posted to your organization's *Joint Commission Connect*® extranet site. A Requirement for Improvement (RFI) in your report means that surveyors found that your organization doesn't comply with a specific standard. All RFIs must be addressed within the time frame listed on the final survey report posted to your organization's *Joint Commission Connect* extranet site. Be aware that 65% of RFIs are given out because an organization doesn't follow its own policy. The Joint Commission may not necessarily require something, but the organization chooses to include something in a policy in an attempt at best practices. If the organization doesn't follow its own policy, it gets an RFI.

Evidence of Standards Compliance

For each RFI, your organization must submit an Evidence of Standards Compliance (ESC) report. There are two types of ESCs:

- **Corrective ESC.** This explains what actions your organization took to bring itself into compliance. The time frame for submitting a corrective ESC is 60 days. It must be done online on an organization's *Joint Commission Connect* extranet site, and it must address the following in detail:
  - **Assigning accountability.** Identify who's ultimately responsible for implementing corrective actions and sustaining compliance.
  - **Correcting noncompliance.** What actions your organization took to correct each finding and when these actions were completed
  - **Ensuring sustained compliance.** A description of the procedures/activities put into place to monitor compliance and details such as the frequency, data collection, and reporting process to ensure sustained compliance
  - **Additional fields.** Under the *SAFER* Matrix, findings determined to be of higher risk and/or broader scope (plotted within the dark orange and red portions of the *SAFER* Matrix) will require organizations to complete two additional fields within their ESC. One of these additional fields includes conducting and documenting a preventive analysis to ensure not only that the noncompliant surface or high-level issue was corrected but also that any underlying reasons for the noncompliance were addressed. In addition, for these higher-risk findings, a description of leadership involvement in bringing the organization into compliance and sustaining compliance is required.

- **Time frame.** All corrective actions must be implemented, and dates noted within the ESC, by the time the ESC is due.

- **Clarification.** This is used when your organization believes it was compliant at the time of the survey. Challenging a surveyor's observation doesn't automatically remove an RFI. You'll need to show proof. This clarification must be submitted within 10 business days following the posting of your organization's final Accreditation Report on the *Joint Commission Connect* site. (Note: An ESC will be due in the same time frame should a clarification not be accepted by The Joint Commission.)

See page 59 for an example of a completed ESC in regard to a hypothetical scenario in which a surveyor cited a hospital under LS.02.01.35, Element of Performance (EP) 4: Piping for approved sprinkler systems is not used to support any other item.

WHY DO I NEED TO KNOW THIS NOW?

The end of the survey process is not really an end. The survey identifies areas for improvement. You need to be ready to address these, as achieving accreditation may depend on you taking corrective action in a limited time frame.

WHERE DO I START?

- **Work with The Joint Commission.** If you are unsure how to address noncompliance issues identified during survey, talk with the surveyor, contact your account executive, or contact the Standards Interpretation Group for advice.
- **Meet with the compliance or performance improvement team.** Although it is not required by the standards that you create a Compliance Committee or a formal performance improvement team, it's a good idea, particularly for larger organizations. The cross-disciplinary expertise available through such groups can be very helpful in resolving compliance problems.

Evidence of Standards Compliance (ESC) Example

Assigning Accountability	Correcting the Non-Compliance	Ensuring Sustained Compliance	All Sections

Assigning Accountability

Instructions
Please indicate, by title, one individual responsible for all corrective actions and ongoing compliance associated with this element of performance. (Note: Even though multiple individuals will likely have a role in the corrective actions, you are asked to identify the one person who has ultimate accountability for the completion of all actions and ongoing compliance.)

The **facilities manager** is ultimately responsible for all corrective actions and ongoing compliance associated with this element of performance.

To keep this Element of Performance on the "To Do" tab, mark this response as In Progress by selected the check box below. This selection will need to be removed prior to submitting the ESC.

□ In Progress

Correcting Non-Compliance

Instructions
Concisely describe the actions completed to correct each finding. This should include policies/procedures developed, revised, and approved. All corrective actions should also include staffing training, communications, and/or spreading awareness. This description must illustrate the finding was fully corrected. (Notes: Do not copy and paste entire policies, bylaws, or other documents in this filed. Even though the corrective actions may encompass multiple dates, please identify the final date that all corrective actions, including education and approvals were completed. The final date entered must be prior to your ESC submission due date and cannot be a future date.)

All corrective actions identified below must be completed prior to submission.

Format ▾ Font ▾ Size ▾ **B** *I* U

As most of the cables resting on the sprinkler piping were installed by our Information Technology (IT) Department and its contractors, Facilities met with IT to work out a solution. Teams from Facilities and IT installed J-hooks in multiple locations throughout the above-ceiling space on the walls well above the sprinkler pipes and ran the cables through the J-hooks rather than letting them continue to rest on the pipes.

The Facilities Department also conducted training sessions for IT, Security, Environmental Services, Construction, Clinical Engineering, and other staff that install equipment or sometimes work above the ceiling, stressing the importance of not letting anything touch the sprinkler piping. To ensure ongoing training, competency, and supervision of staff and any outside contractor workers who enter that space, the hospital implemented an above-ceiling permit policy. Anyone needing access to the space above the ceiling must apply for a permit, which requires reading the policy and procedures and signing an attestation that these have been read and understood. The permit must be displayed on the ladder being used by anyone working above the ceiling. For outside contractors and staff in departments other than Facilities, any work performed above the ceiling must be inspected and signed off by a designated Facilities supervisor.

Format ▾ Font ▾ Size ▾ B I U

All corrective actions describe above were completed by <u>February 24, 2023</u>.

To keep this Element of Performance on the "To Do" tab, mark this response as In Progress by selecting the check box below. This selection will need to be removed prior to submitting the EST or POC.

☐ In Progress

Ensuring Sustained Compliance

Instructions

While correcting the noncompliant issue is important, the organization should also have a plan for ensuring and sustaining compliance with the Element of Performance across the organization. To support sustainment, a strong strategy to monitor compliance must be developed and implemented. Please use the area below to describe your plan for monitoring future compliance.

What procedures or activities have been identified to monitor your compliance with this Element of Performance?

Format ▾ Font ▾ Size ▾ B I U

Above-ceiling inspection has been incorporated into the hospital's quarterly environmental tours and the annual internal *Life Safety Code® Building Assessment. In addition, as stated above, the hospital's new above-ceiling permit process requires inspection of any work done by outside contractors and non-Facilities staff above the ceiling. Pertinent staff's knowledge of the need to keep anything from touching sprinkler pipes and the above-ceiling permit policy is assessed and documented during training for new staff and biannual refresher training sessions, as well as when a staff member requests a permit to go above the ceiling.**

With any new construction or remodeling, the above-ceiling space will receive added attention to make sure that enough J-hooks or similar devices are included from the onset to facilitate the running of cables and wires.

Format ▾ Font ▾ Size ▾ B I U

What is the frequency of the monitoring activities?

Format ▾ Font ▾ Size ▾ B I U

As stated previously, above-ceiling inspections to make sure cables and wires are not touching sprinkler pipes (as well as other potential issues) are conducted during quarterly environmental tours, the annual internal Building Assessment, and whenever work is performed above the ceiling.

---

* *Life Safety Code®* is a registered trademark of the National Fire Protection Association, Quincy, MA.

Format · Font · Size · B I U

What data will be collected from these activities?

Format · Font · Size · B I U

Data will be collected on who receives training that covers sprinkler system integrity and the competency assessments of those individuals. In addition, the hospital will collect data regarding who applies for above-ceiling permits and the results of the inspections after the work is finished. Moreover, the hospital will gather data on whether any deficiencies are found under LS.02.01.35, EP 4, during quarterly environmental tours and the annual internal Building Inspection.

Format · Font · Size · B I U

To whom, and how often, will this data be reported?

Format · Font · Size · B I U

This data will be reported during monthly Environment of Care Committee meetings and quarterly to the Vice President of Facilities. If the data do not show compliance improvement, the hospital will reassess its training, inspection, and above-ceiling permit processes.

KEY CONCEPT

ACCREDITATION OUTCOMES

As stated previously, accreditation is not necessarily a pass/fail decision. The initial survey is an evaluation of how well you are complying with standards and elements of performance (EPs), and not being fully compliant doesn't mean you will be turned down. The Joint Commission may require your organization to take some specific corrective actions on the way to compliance.

Possible Decision Outcomes

The scoring and decision process is based on an evaluation of compliance with Joint Commission standards and other requirements. Compliance with the standards is scored according to specific performance expectations—the EPs. At the end of the on-site survey, a "Summary of Survey Findings Report" is left with the organization to identify any Requirements for Improvement (RFIs). Organizations with RFIs will have a set period of time to work directly with their account executive to submit evidence to show that the organization is now in full compliance with those standards.

- **Accreditation** is awarded to a health care organization that complies with all applicable standards at the time of the survey or has successfully addressed all RFIs in an ESC submission within 60 days following the posting of the Accreditation Survey Findings Report and does not meet any other rules for other accreditation decisions.

"I heard that...

patient care standards relate only to inpatients and individuals being served in health care facilities."

fact:

Caring for an individual doesn't stop at the door of your facility. For instance, in the case of some addiction treatment programs, standards cover how organizations handle individuals who cannot immediately be placed in an inpatient setting. Joint Commission standards across programs require educating individuals receiving care and their families about self-care and discharge plans. Standards also require organizations to assess, refer, and report cases of potential abuse and neglect, even if the reason for a visit is unrelated to the abuse or neglect.

"I heard that...

there's a certain number of findings a surveyor can note that will automatically lead to Denial of Accreditation."

fact:

Your surveyor does not render a decision at the time of survey. In addition, there's no specific number of findings that will trigger denial (although there are types of triggers, such as unlicensed physicians, that can lead to a denial). Denial of Accreditation is recommended in very specific circumstances: The organization doesn't permit The Joint Commission to perform a survey; the organization failed to resolve certain statuses before withdrawing from the accreditation process; the organization failed to submit payment for survey fees; and the organization repeatedly failed to submit an ESC. *See* the ACC chapter on E-dition or in the *Comprehensive Accreditation Manual* for details.

- **Accreditation with Follow-up Survey** results when a health care organization complies with all standards, as determined by an acceptable ESC submission. A follow-up survey is required within six months to assess sustained compliance.
- **Limited, Temporary Accreditation** results when a health care organization is in satisfactory compliance with the limited set of standards and EPs assessed in the first of the two surveys conducted under the Early Survey Policy (ESP).
- **Preliminary Denial of Accreditation** is recommended when there is justification to deny accreditation to a health care organization as evidenced by one or more of the following: an Immediate Threat to Health or Safety to care recipients or the public; submission of falsified documents or misrepresented information; lack of a required license or similar issue at the time of survey; failure to resolve the requirements of an Accreditation with Follow-up Survey status; or significant noncompliance with Joint Commission standards. This decision may be subject to review and appeal by the organization before the determination to deny accreditation.
- **Denial of Accreditation** results when a health care organization has been denied accreditation. All review and appeal opportunities have been exhausted. For an organization undergoing an initial survey, the organization has failed to demonstrate compliance with all applicable Joint Commission standards.

Accreditation Effective Dates and Duration

In most situations, accreditation is valid for three years from the last day of survey. Laboratory accreditation is good for two years. If you opt for the ESP (*see* Chapter 3), the accreditation is effective the day after your second survey if you receive no RFIs. If you do receive RFIs, your accreditation will become effective as soon as you submit an acceptable ESC.

Accreditation Award Display and Use

When you have been awarded accreditation by The Joint Commission, your organization is entitled to display The Joint Commission's Gold Seal of Approval®. The Joint Commission website features a publicity kit that covers the ins and outs of how and where you may display the award. And the following list contains some suggestions for displaying and celebrating your accreditation:

- Use the Gold Seal of Approval to promote your organization's Joint Commission accreditation. Gold Seal of Approval decals are available to download for your organization to display at the main entrance of the facility. Your organization can download artwork of the Gold Seal of Approval from our online publicity kit to incorporate the Gold Seal of Approval into print, billboard, television, and online advertising; letterhead and stationery; business cards; educational materials for care recipients; and your organization's website.
- Your organization can also order Gold Seal of Approval products through our affiliate, JCR. Visit the JCR store at **https://www.jcrinc.com/** or call JCR Customer Service toll-free at (877) 223-6866.
- Display your organization's Certificate of Accreditation in a prominent location(s) in your organization. To order additional certificates call (630) 792-5871.
- Print and distribute the brochure *We Achieved The Gold Seal of Approval® from The Joint Commission* (*see* "Recommended Resources" for a link to the publicity kit) to explain to your care recipients and community that

PICTURE THIS

The Gold Seal of Approval®

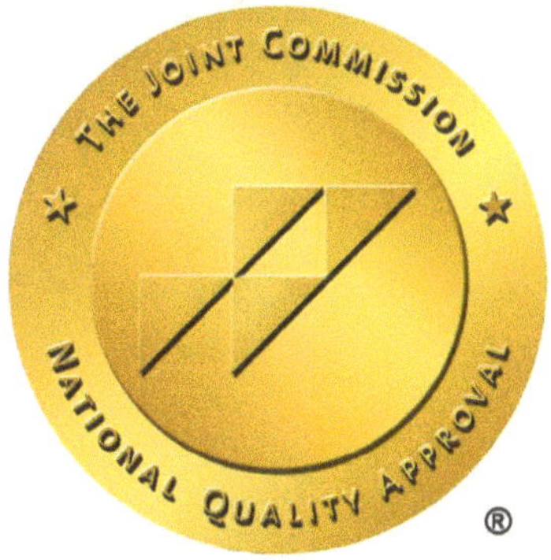

The Joint Commission offers its Gold Seal of Approval® to accredited organizations in recognition of their efforts to provide high-quality care, treatment, and services. Organizations receive and can display the Gold Seal when they have successfully completed their accreditation survey under the full set of standards (including the second survey in the Early Survey Policy).

accreditation, certification, and verification signify that your organization meets rigorous performance standards in delivering high-quality, safe care.

- Send a news release to the local media. *See* the sample news releases in the publicity kit.
- Conduct a news conference. Invite local reporters to meet with your organization's CEO, medical director, quality assurance/improvement director, and other key staff members. Discuss how staff involvement is essential to both maintaining continuous standards compliance and demonstrating that compliance during the unannounced survey. Explain the focus on the care, treatment, and services of care recipients through the tracer methodology and observation of care. Emphasize how the survey is tailored to your organization's unique characteristics, services, and care recipient populations. Stress your organization's ongoing continuous compliance with standards 24/7, 365 days a year.
- Demonstrate ongoing efforts to comply with Joint Commission standards that can provide additional positive publicity. For example, invite the news media to cover emergency drills. This is a highly visible, graphic story and generates positive media exposure. Discuss individual tracers and the wide range of standards on which your organization was evaluated.

TOOL

News Release Template

- Notify any state or metropolitan provider association of which your organization is a member. Many of these associations publicize accreditation information in their newsletters.
- Notify the benefits manager at insurance carriers and/or health plans whose clients use or might use your organization's services.
- Include information on the benefits of accreditation in your organization's newsletters and in presentations to staff, board members, and community groups.
- Celebrate the accreditation award by sponsoring a "Quality Day" at your organization. Honor special staff, volunteers, or donors and offer tours of your organization's facility.

WHY DO I NEED TO KNOW THIS NOW?

After preparing for and participating in a Joint Commission survey, it's important to know what the outcome may be and how to announce your new or renewed accreditation status.

WHERE DO I START?

- **Talk with Joint Commission surveyors.** Before they depart, talk with the Joint Commission surveyors to ensure that you know the next steps.
- **Review the Final Accreditation Report.** When completed, the Final Accreditation Report will be posted to your *Joint Commission Connect* extranet site. Contact your account executive with any questions you may have before receiving it or after you have reviewed it.

Test Your Knowledge

1. What are the findings on a Joint Commission accreditation survey report called?
   - ☐ a. Observations
   - ☐ b. Deficiencies
   - ☐ c. Requirements for improvement
   - ☐ d. Recommendations
2. The *Survey Analysis for Evaluating Risk®* Matrix determines your organization's accreditation decision.
   - ☐ a. True
   - ☐ b. False
3. When responding to items listed on a Joint Commission accreditation survey report, the response is called ___________.
   - ☐ a. a Plan of Correction
   - ☐ b. Evidence of Standards Compliance
   - ☐ c. a Corrective Action Plan
   - ☐ d. Proof of Resolution
4. Your organization receives its final accreditation report. Leaders disagree with two items on the report. The next two questions are based on this scenario.

   4A. If your organization wishes to challenge the two items, this is called a(n) ___________.
   - ☐ a. appeal
   - ☐ b. challenge
   - ☐ c. clarification
   - ☐ d. reconsideration

   4B. Within how many business days after you receive your report must you file the challenge?
   - ☐ a. 5
   - ☐ b. 10
   - ☐ c. 15
   - ☐ d. 30
5. Joint Commission accreditation is valid for three years, with the exception of one program. Which program is this?
   - ☐ a. Ambulatory Care
   - ☐ b. Laboratory and Point-of-Care Testing
   - ☐ c. Nursing Care Center
   - ☐ d. Health Care Staffing

(continued)

(continued)

6. During an accreditation survey, a serious safety issue (such as finding that several surgical instruments used in surgery had no proof of proper sterilization over several weeks) was identified. The next questions are based on this scenario.

6A. Which of the following is The Joint Commission's term for this situation?

- ☐ a. Immediate Jeopardy
- ☐ b. Immediate Threat to Life
- ☐ c. Immediate Threat to Health and Safety

6B. Which of the following could be the accreditation decision for this organization?

- ☐ a. Preliminary Denial of Accreditation
- ☐ b. CMS-2567 Plan of Action
- ☐ c. Partial Accreditation

Maintaining Your Accreditation Compliance

CHAPTER 6

THE BIG IDEA

Now that you have achieved Joint Commission accreditation, you will need to ensure that your organization continues to comply with standards and elements of performance (EPs), not to mention providing safe, effective, and high-quality care and treatment to care recipients. In this chapter we will discuss strategies and provide tools for maintaining accreditation.

KEY CONCEPTS

- Continuous Compliance
- Sentinel Event Follow-Up
- Organizational Changes and Accreditation
- Maintaining Safety by Staying Informed

THE MANUAL

Following is the relevant Joint Commission E-dition® or *Comprehensive Accreditation Manual* chapter:

- "The Accreditation Process" (ACC)

KEY CONCEPT

CONTINUOUS COMPLIANCE

This is what it's all about: maintaining continuous compliance. This is how your organization will shine—as bright as the Joint Commission Gold Seal of Approval®. It takes a lot of work on your part, and The Joint Commission is there to work with you.

Intracycle Monitoring (ICM) Profile

The Joint Commission offers a suite of tools to help you maintain compliance between surveys: the Intracycle Monitoring (ICM) Profile. Through your secure *Joint Commission Connect®* extranet site, you can access your organization's ICM Profile. The profile includes your accreditation status information, major risk areas, and resources. You also may request an ICM survey in which you pick the team and the length of time the survey team is on site. This provides an opportunity for a team of actual Joint Commission surveyors to pre-identify any potential areas of noncompliance.

Focused Standards Assessment (FSA)

One major component of the ICM Profile is the Focused Standards Assessment (FSA). Your accredited organization may complete this self-assessment activity between Joint Commission surveys to help maintain compliance. It scores the same way surveyors do during a survey, identifies areas of noncompliance, and requires a Plan of Action (POA) for any Requirement for Improvement (RFI). (In certain instances, your organization may be required to complete the FSA. You will be notified if this is the case.)

Impact of the FSA on accreditation. The FSA doesn't affect your organization's accreditation status unless when completing it you identify an Immediate Threat to Health or Safety and a special survey is conducted.

Completing the FSA. You can complete the FSA in one of the following ways:

- **Full FSA**
  - Use the automated tool to assess and score compliance.
  - Create a POA for every area of noncompliance and submit it to The Joint Commission.
- **Option 1 (Attestation)**
  - Use the FSA tool or alternative methodology to assess compliance.
  - Inform The Joint Commission that you completed the assessment and have developed POAs, but don't submit standard scoring.
- **Option 2 (ICM survey, written documentation of findings)**
  - Request and participate in an educational survey (a fee is charged for this survey).
  - Receive a written report of survey findings; review and submit relevant POA to The Joint Commission.
  - Discuss any issues with Joint Commission staff via telephone, if desired.

- **Option 3 (ICM survey, oral exit briefing)**
  - Request and participate in an educational survey (a fee is charged for this survey).
  - Receive an oral report of findings at the end of the survey.
  - No written report will be left at the organization, and no findings are transmitted to The Joint Commission.

Mock Tracers

You can perform tracers within your organization just like Joint Commission surveyors do. They are a great way of evaluating how well the organization is providing care, treatment, and services and how well you are complying with Joint Commission standards and EPs. Mock tracers have the added benefit of getting and keeping staff comfortable and engaged with continuous compliance and the tracer process, which helps things go more smoothly at survey time.

PICTURE THIS

The Accreditation Cycle

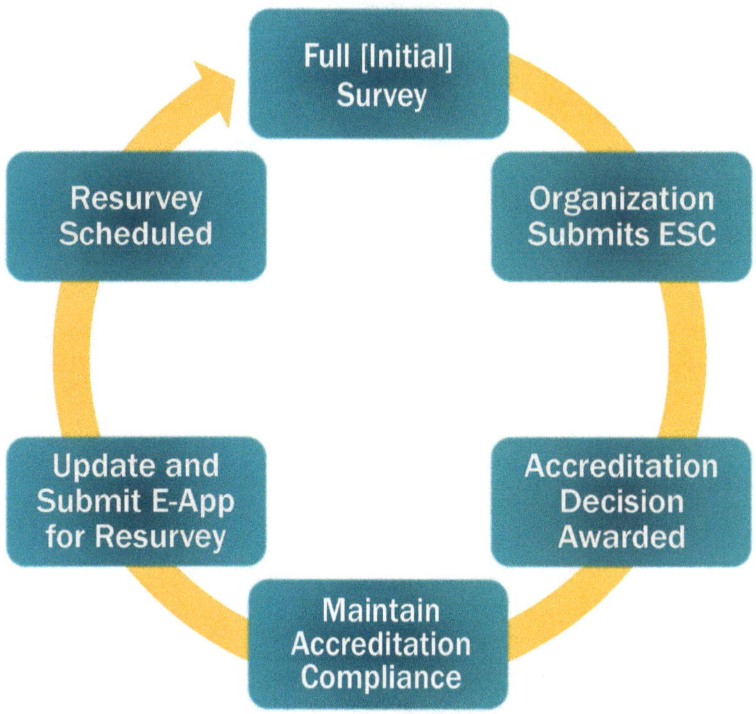
Full [Initial] Survey
Organization Submits ESC
Accreditation Decision Awarded
Maintain Accreditation Compliance
Update and Submit E-App for Resurvey
Resurvey Scheduled

Preparing for your first survey may seem overwhelming and complicated, but the accreditation cycle itself is simple and straightforward. After your organization completes and submits its electronic application for accreditation (E-App) and deposit, access to your secure *Joint Commission Connect* extranet site, which includes access to E-dition, is available.

ESC, Evidence of Standards Compliance.

As with tracers conducted during a survey, you may choose to conduct an individual tracer, in which you follow a care recipient through their entire course of care, or a system tracer, in which you take an in-depth look at a specific program, process, or system to evaluate how well it is working.

There are 10 essential steps to conducting a mock tracer, and these can be broken down into four phases:

- **Phase 1.** Planning and Preparing
  1. **Establish a schedule.** It should be clear to everyone how long the process is going to take and when to expect results.
  2. **Determine the scope.** Decide whether you will conduct an individual or system tracer and, if it's the latter, decide which system to focus on.
  3. **Choose mock surveyors.** Choose who will conduct the tracer based on their expertise in the system you are surveying or their background in the area of treatment and services being provided to the subject.
  4. **Train mock surveyors.** Mock surveyors may need to interact with care recipients and their families, clinicians, nurses, laboratory staff, security personnel, front desk staff, or others, depending on the scope of your tracer. Let them know what data and information you are looking for and how best to go about obtaining them.
- **Phase 2.** Conducting and Evaluating
  5. **Assign the mock tracer.** Match experts to subjects.
  6. **Conduct the mock tracer.** Send your mock surveyors out to collect data and information from documentation, observation of processes, and interviews.
  7. **Debrief about the process.** Hold an open forum where mock surveyors can present their findings. Let your tracer team give feedback on the process to help you conduct more tracers in the future.
- **Phase 3.** Analyzing and Reporting
  8. **Analyze the data.** Organize your data to help you and your team draw conclusions about what you have observed. What are you doing well? What could be improved and how?
  9. **Report your results.** Present your results as a panel and post them for feedback. Highlight what you are doing well and be clear about what needs improvement.
- **Phase 4.** Apply the Results
  10. **Develop and implement plans for improvement.** Based on the results of your mock tracer, develop plans for improvement that have specific goals, measures for improvement, and well-defined time frames that allow you to assess whether performance is, in fact, improving and improvements are sustained.

TOOLS

Mock Tracer Form

Mock Tracer Planning Task List

Mock Tracer Evaluation Checklist

See "Recommended Resources" near the end of this book for some suggested resources for conducting mock tracers and making the most of them.

WHY DO I NEED TO KNOW THIS NOW?

Continuous compliance is the goal. The ICM Profile is a set of tools to help you meet that goal. If you learn about it now, you'll be better able to use it to keep your organization on track and reduce RFIs in the survey.

WHERE DO I START?

- **Review documents.** If your organization is already accredited, log in to your *Joint Commission Connect* extranet site and review the status of your FSA. If required or desired, either complete the full FSA or request one of the other three options.
- **Conduct tracers.** EPs that fall under FSA risk categories differ for each accreditation program. Become familiar with those for your organization's program setting. They make good candidates for focused, or spot, mock tracers on problem areas in your organization. Reminder: If a standard includes one or more EPs with an R, all EPs under that standard should be scored to meet FSA expectations.
- **Be a role model.** If you want to involve leaders in continuous compliance and survey readiness, be prepared to show them ways to do that. Department by department. Leader by leader. One way to do this is with a daily sweep, which you can encourage by volunteering to do it periodically in each department.

KEY CONCEPT

SENTINEL EVENT FOLLOW-UP

All sentinel events (as defined in Chapter 1 on page 12 and explored in greater detail in the "Sentinel Event Policy" [SE] chapter on E-dition or in your *Comprehensive Accreditation Manual*) must be reviewed by an organization, whether or not they are reported to The Joint Commission. The organization must complete a thorough comprehensive systematic analysis (most commonly a root cause analysis) to determine why the event occurred. The organization must then create a corrective action plan to prevent similar events from happening, implement the plan, and monitor its effectiveness.

The Joint Commission's Office of Quality and Patient Safety will conduct a collaborative review with organization leaders or a designee to determine whether the comprehensive systematic analysis and corrective action plan are acceptable.

The fact that an organization experienced a sentinel event will not affect its accreditation decision. However, willful failure to respond appropriately to the sentinel event could have an impact. In these instances, safety specialists in The Joint Commission's Office of Quality and Patient Safety, along with the Joint Commission medical director and patient safety officer, would recommend to the executive leaders of The Joint Commission and the Accreditation Council to revise the organization's accreditation status.

Sentinel Event Alerts and Performance Improvement

The Joint Commission periodically publishes *Sentinel Event Alerts* addressing high-priority safety and/or care issues that apply to a significant number of accredited organizations. *Sentinel Event Alerts* are not surveyable, but they may be sources for performance improvement (PI) initiatives. Each *Sentinel Event Alert* does the following:

- Identifies specific types of sentinel events
- Describes their common underlying causes
- Suggests steps to prevent future occurrences

WHY DO I NEED TO KNOW THIS NOW?

You can't get started on improvements until you have a plan to identify PI opportunities and address them. Setting priorities is part of Joint Commission Performance Improvement (PI) standards, as well as its Leadership (LD) standards.

WHERE DO I START?

- **Review documents.** As a new accreditation manager, ask to review any PI plans. Look for the following:
  - All required data collection and reporting processes
  - Relevant analyses and action plans
  - Time frames for each plan to reflect priorities
- **Facilitate processes.** If your organization doesn't already have a standardized method for prioritizing PI projects, make that a priority. Some organizations use a coding system.
- **Work with leaders.** Show leaders that you want to—and need to—know about PI opportunities.
  - Review *Sentinel Event Alerts* for potential applicability to your organization. Share the information with the PI team and leaders. Then together identify which recommendations (if any) from the *Sentinel Event Alert* you should consider for implementation.
  - Suggest using WalkRounds™ (*see* Chapter 16) or other similar approaches to encourage leaders to get out on the front line and engage with staff about potential PI project opportunities.

KEY CONCEPT

ORGANIZATIONAL CHANGES AND ACCREDITATION

Change is a given. Health care organizations open new facilities and close others. Some expand services. Contractual relationships change. Unforeseen events change the organization's ability to fulfill its function. You are required to report certain kinds of organizational changes to The Joint Commission within 30 days. These include the following:

- Change of ownership or control
- Change of location
- Change of capacity
- Change of services offered

For deemed status. Any organization using Joint Commission accreditation for deemed status must notify The Joint Commission immediately if it receives a notice from a regulatory agency, such as the US Centers for Medicare & Medicaid Services (CMS), that its deemed status has been removed due to noncompliance identified during a recent complaint or validation survey.

Accreditation Status After a Disaster

Following a disaster that requires a Joint Commission–accredited organization to cease the provision of services for a period of time, The Joint Commission will work with the affected organization to address the impact that the cessation of services will have on the organization's accreditation status and to ensure that the organization is prepared to provide safe, high-quality care upon resumption of services. If after six months the organization cannot resume services, The Joint Commission will discontinue the accreditation of the organization. The impact of the cessation of services for a period of time on the accreditation status of organizations that experience a disaster is described below.

- **Cease services up to 30 days.** For organizations that resume services within the first 30 days after a disaster and/or the organization's decision to cease operations, the organization's original Joint Commission accreditation status will stay in effect. The time frame for complying with any outstanding Joint Commission requirements (such as Evidence of Standards Compliance [ESC]) will pause until the organization resumes operation. In most cases, The Joint Commission will not need to survey the affected organization to reassess its level of standards compliance. If The Joint Commission decides to conduct a survey, however, the organization's accreditation decision will be driven by the interim survey findings.

- **Cease services up to 90 days.** For organizations that resume services from 31 to 90 days after a disaster, The Joint Commission will conduct an extension survey to determine the organization's accreditation status. The circumstances surrounding the organization's closure will determine the survey's length and scope.

- **Cease services up to six months.** For organizations that resume services from 91 days up to six months after a disaster, The Joint Commission will require a survey to assess the environment of care (if applicable). This survey will preferably take place one to two weeks after services are resumed. These organizations must receive clearance to operate from the fire marshal, if appropriate, and other local/state authorities before resuming services. In addition, The Joint Commission will conduct a second survey approximately four months after services have been resumed to evaluate sustained compliance with Joint Commission standards and requirements. The track record requirement for demonstrating standards compliance will be four months.

- **More than six months.** For organizations that do not resume services within six months after a disaster or decide to cease operations, The Joint Commission will discontinue its accreditation. If the organization resumes services, it must reapply to become accredited. In such cases, the accreditation process will involve at least two surveys. The first survey will be conducted at the organization's request and will assess the organization's ability to provide safe care to individuals. The organization may qualify for an accreditation award as a result of this survey. However, at this point, the organization will not be recognized by CMS as meeting the requirements for

Medicare certification and may not be recognized by any other regulatory agency from which the organization receives deemed status. The second survey will be conducted approximately four months later to assess sustained compliance with Joint Commission requirements. The track record requirement for demonstrating standards compliance will be four months.

Accreditation Status When Services Have Ceased

Joint Commission–accredited organizations may stop providing care, treatment, and services or may not provide health care or services to care recipients for a period of time for reasons other than natural or human-made disasters. When a health care organization ceases to provide care services, it is required to notify The Joint Commission. The Joint Commission will work with the affected organization to address the impact that the cessation of services or the lack of care recipients will have on the organization's accreditation status and to ensure that the organization is prepared to provide safe, high-quality care, treatment, or services upon resumption of services. If after six months the organization cannot resume services, The Joint Commission will terminate the accreditation of the organization.

- **Up to 60 days.** If an organization does not have any care recipients for up to 60 days, The Joint Commission will continue the organization's current accreditation status.
- **Up to six months.** If an organization does not have any care recipients from 60 days to less than six months, but then resumes services within six months, The Joint Commission will continue the organization's current accreditation status only if the organization has an extension survey. This extension survey would generally take place as soon as possible in accordance with the organization's request. The purpose of this survey is to evaluate the organization's capability for resuming services and whether it is performing at current accreditation levels. If the organization refuses an extension survey, the accreditation will be terminated.
- **More than six months.** If an organization does not have any care recipients for six months or longer, The Joint Commission will terminate the organization's accreditation. If the organization resumes services, it will have to reapply for accreditation and have a full survey to evaluate its current compliance with Joint Commission standards.

WHY DO I NEED TO KNOW THIS NOW?

After a disaster or cessation of services, the organization will want to get back up and running as soon as it can and to assure the public that it is able to provide care, treatment, and services in a safe environment.

WHERE DO I START?

- **Learn more.** Familiarize yourself with emergency management procedures, particularly regarding recovery after an emergency. Also, because a disaster may affect facilities, you should familiarize yourself with the requirements of the "Life Safety" (LS) chapter on E-dition or in the *Comprehensive Accreditation Manual* as well as the *Life Safety Code*®* published by the National Fire Protection Association.

---

* *Life Safety Code*® is a registered trademark of the National Fire Protection Association, Quincy, MA.

- **Reach out to experts.** In the wake of a disaster you will need to work with the fire marshal, structural engineers, and others to ensure that your facilities are safe to occupy. Try reaching out to these people beforehand to develop a working relationship in advance of need.

KEY CONCEPT

MAINTAINING SAFETY BY STAYING INFORMED

In addition to twice-annual updates to the accreditation standards, The Joint Commission is continuously reviewing and updating its policies and recommendations based on research, client feedback, and evolving best practices. You can stay abreast of these developments by using a number of digital resources provided by The Joint Commission and Joint Commission Resources.

Maintaining Safety

The Joint Commission offers tools to help you maintain safety and stay abreast of developments in safety research and practice.

Among the useful tools and information The Joint Commission offers are the following:

Quick Safety. *Quick Safety* is an alert published by The Joint Commission that covers an incident or a trend in care recipient or worker safety. Past issues have covered topics such as severe pressure injuries; pregnancy-related death; and preventing light source–related burns from laparoscopy, thoracoscopy, and arthroscopy; just to name a few.

Sentinel Event Alerts. From time to time sentinel event data and other data analyzed by Joint Commission professionals suggest trends in certain serious safety incidents. When this happens, The Joint Commission publishes a *Sentinel Event Alert*. These alerts are a way of informing those in the health care industry of emerging safety trends affecting the individuals they serve, giving them reliable information about those trends, and providing evidence-based tools and strategies for preventing certain kinds of sentinel events. Previous *Sentinel Event Alerts* have covered such topics as surgical fire prevention, preserving patient safety after a cyberattack, and eliminating disparities for pregnant patients.

Perspectives

Joint Commission Perspectives® provides authoritative, accurate, and timely information about revisions and updates to Joint Commission standards, policies, and other requirements for all Joint Commission–accredited, –certified, and –verified organizations. *Perspectives* is published monthly and covers all accredited and certified health care settings.

All Joint Commission–accredited, –certified, and –verified organizations receive complimentary access via their secure *Joint Commission Connect* extranet site and may share the newsletter within the organization. To further ensure that staff in your organization are up to date on any Joint Commission requirement and/or survey process changes, all staff in your organization may access *Perspectives* by signing up for "Guest Access" to *Joint Commission Connect*. This expanded access ensures that staff throughout your organization will be informed whether or not they have full access to your *Joint Commission Connect* extranet site.

Joint Commission Connect

Joint Commission Connect is a secure extranet website to The Joint Commission. It is the portal through which accredited, certified, and verified health care organizations interact with The Joint Commission. *Joint Commission Connect* is where you submit your application and other documentation required by The Joint Commission, and it is gateway to a wealth of essential information about updates to standards, standards application guidance, and everything related to your accreditation, certification, and verification status and activities.

Make sure to identify at least one person to be your *Joint Commission Connect* security administrator. This person will manage the organization's *Joint Commission Connect* account, login credentials, and other administrative issues. Be sure to update the contact information for your account administrator regularly so your account executive knows whom to contact regarding any problem regarding the site or access to it.

Joint Commission Newsletters/E-Alerts/Blogs

Joint Commission Online. Published each Wednesday, *Joint Commission Online* reports news about Joint Commission standards, the survey process, patient safety, and more.

Program-specific blogs/newsletters. The Joint Commission also publishes a variety of program-specific blogs, newsletters, and e-alerts that any staff may sign up for on The Joint Commission's website. Access to your organization's *Joint Commission Connect* extranet site is not needed.

Patient Safety Topics. Located on The Joint Commission's website under Resources, these patient safety topics portals offer a collection of resources on the following topics:

- Zero Harm
- Emergency Management
- Health Care Workforce Safety and Well-Being
- Infection Prevention and Control
- Report a Patient Safety Concern or Complaint
- Suicide Prevention
- Workplace Violence Prevention

Visit The Joint Commission's website to sign up for alerts, blog posts, and newsletters.

WHY DO I NEED TO KNOW THIS NOW?

To provide high-quality care, treatment, and services in a safe environment, it is important to remain up to date on news and changes from The Joint Commission.

Test Your Knowledge

1. If you are Joint Commission accredited and choose to use the Focused Standards Assessment (FSA), how often must you typically complete it?
   - ☐ a. Twice a year
   - ☐ b. Annually
   - ☐ c. Between triennial surveys
   - ☐ d. Never
2. Do Joint Commission surveyors have access to completed FSAs?
   - ☐ a. Yes
   - ☐ b. No
3. You receive a report that part of a surgical sponge was left inside a patient who had emergency life-saving surgery after an automobile crash. A surgeon had to operate the day after the original surgery to remove it. The patient is doing well and gives rave reviews on social media for the surgeons and staff. Which of the following would best describe the situation in Joint Commission terminology?
   - ☐ a. A surgical error
   - ☐ b. A close call
   - ☐ c. A sentinel event
4. Which of the following could be considered examples of a mock survey? (Select all that apply.)
   - ☐ a. Practice session at the end of the quality committee meeting
   - ☐ b. External consultants conducting time-out observations
   - ☐ c. Chart review with the treatment team
   - ☐ d. Leadership rounding
5. Which of the following is the official Joint Commission newsletter for accreditation, certification, and verification compliance?
   - ☐ a. E-dition®
   - ☐ b. *Quick Safety*
   - ☐ c. *Perspectives*

PART 3
Understanding Joint Commission–Related Data

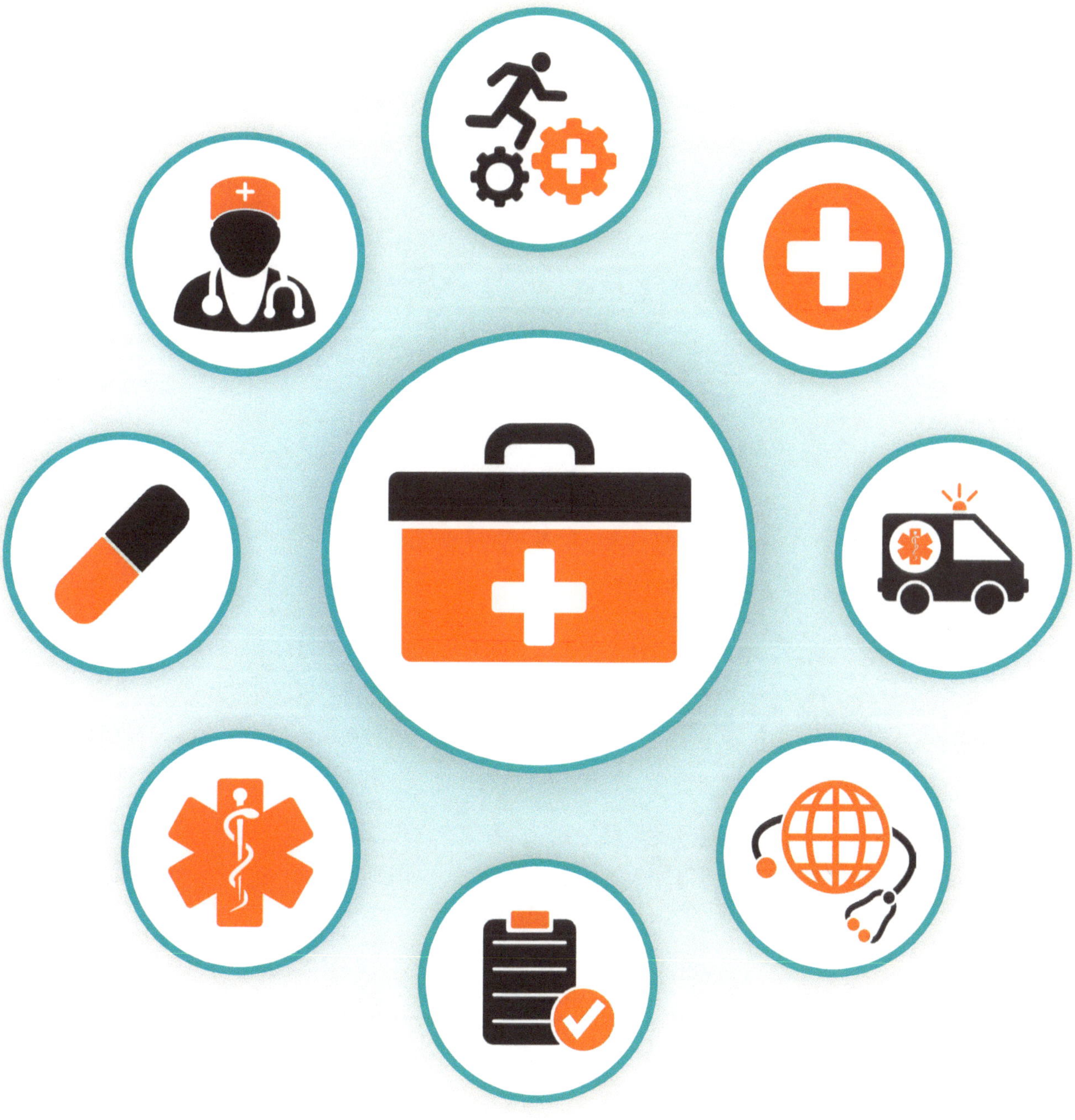

Performance Measures and The Joint Commission

CHAPTER 7

THE BIG IDEA

In its ongoing mission to improve the quality of health care, The Joint Commission has various quality and performance measures reporting requirements. Some accreditation programs have select measures that are part of Accreditation Participation Requirements. In addition, although not addressed in this *Toolkit*, many Joint Commission certification/verification programs and advanced disease-specific care certification programs specify select measures as part of certification/verification participation requirements. Regulatory agencies—such as the US Centers for Medicare & Medicaid Services (CMS)—may use quality reporting programs that your organization also must comply with. Where possible, The Joint Commission and regulatory agencies have worked together to closely align their measures and reporting requirements to streamline data collection reporting, which eliminates duplicative work for your organization. Of course, your organization is likely to use other measures internally for performance monitoring and improvement activities.

How do you know a good measure from one that doesn't provide meaningful data? In this chapter we will look at different kinds of performance measures and the requirements for creating sound and useful measures.

KEY CONCEPTS

- Constructing Measures
- Accountability Measures
- ORYX® Measures

THE MANUAL

Following are the relevant Joint Commission E-dition® or *Comprehensive Accreditation Manual* chapters:

- "Accreditation Participation Requirements" (APR)
- "Information Management" (IM)
- "National Patient Safety Goals" (NPSG)
- "Performance Improvement" (PI)
- "Performance Measurement and the ORYX Initiative" (PM) [assisted living community, critical access hospital, and hospital only]

KEY CONCEPT

CONSTRUCTING MEASURES

A great deal of research has been and is being done into the design and vetting of credible evidence-based measures of the quality of care. Several challenges arise in construction, including understanding how best to collect data. For example, do claims data and 30-day mortality statistics meaningfully measure how well the organization is performing a process or function? Or are they too far downstream to provide meaningful information? Do certain kinds of reporting lead to "gaming" of the system? These are important considerations when deciding what to measure and how.

The Joint Commission works continuously to develop and evolve meaningful measures of health care performance through research and collaboration with regulatory agencies and health care quality organizations. Chapter 8 will explore the various data collection and reporting requirements you may encounter. In this chapter we will provide you a broad overview of performance measures, what makes a good one, and what the pitfalls can be.

Types of Measures

The Joint Commission is a leader in the development of performance measures for health care organizations. Since the 1980s The Joint Commission has spearheaded numerous initiatives to develop, test, and implement meaningful performance measures that health care organizations use for performance improvement (PI) activities, as part of the data they provide at survey, and for public reporting purposes. Measure development initiatives undertaken at The Joint Commission led to developing performance measures for stroke, maternal care, perinatal care, venous thromboembolism, heart attack care, and hospital-based inpatient psychiatric services (HBIPS).

To effectively construct measures, you need to understand the types of measures you will be working with. The broad performance measure categories you will be working with include the following:

- **Process measures.** Process measures are used to assess a goal-directed, interrelated series of actions, events, mechanisms, or steps—such as a measure of performance that describes what is done to, for, or by individuals receiving care. For example, tracking the percentage of individuals receiving care who receive immunizations is a process measure.
- **Outcome measures.** Outcome measures indicate the results of performance (or nonperformance) of a function(s) or process(es). For example, surgical site infections related to abdominal hysterectomy is an outcome measure.
- **Continuous variable measures.** An aggregate data measure in which the value of each measurement can fall anywhere along a continuous scale (for example, the time [in minutes] from hospital arrival to administration of thrombolysis).

Each of these categories has its advantages for certain kinds of investigations. Some measures will, of course, be dictated by the requirements of The Joint Commission and/or regulatory agencies used for quality reporting, but in your own PI initiatives, using a mix of these measure types will be most effective. This will help you get a balanced view of baseline performance and the effect of PI projects.

WHY DO I NEED TO KNOW THIS NOW?

Bad performance measures can be worse than useless. They can lead to adverse outcomes, wasted effort, and a false sense of security.

WHERE DO I START?

- **Learn more.** The Joint Commission and the federal government are both dedicated to developing and disseminating the best possible quality measures for health care. Both publish papers and other information about quality measure development. Visit The Joint Commission's website and explore the "Measurement" section. There you will find a wealth of information on Joint Commission reporting requirements and how to meet them. Familiarize yourself with the principles of what makes good quality measures for your specific setting.
- **Encourage technology use.** As the industry transitions away from paper records to electronic health records (EHRs), so too does it transition away from "chart-abstracted" data. In the past, staff at health care organizations would pore over health records and compile the health care data therein. As time goes on, both The Joint Commission and regulatory agencies are relying more on processes that automatically extract data from the EHR, which saves time and money, facilitates standardization of data and measures, and increases reporting rates and accuracy.
- **Facilitate processes.** Integrate performance measurement and reporting into your organizationwide PI program. Measures should be developed with evidence-based guidelines to ensure that solid measures are being used that fit your organization's reporting needs and circumstances.

"I heard that...

deemed organizations that do not meet reporting requirements set by CMS can be hit with financial penalties."

fact

The Joint Commission strives to align—where possible—the data submission requirements with CMS. The data are submitted separately, but the reporting requirements are similar for both organizations. In its desire to reward organizations that produce better health outcomes, CMS has embedded standardized measures in several quality reporting programs. Within the CMS quality reporting programs, the results of the measures may affect payment and/or incentives to organizations. The Joint Commission uses the measures for quality improvement purposes.

KEY CONCEPT

ACCOUNTABILITY MEASURES

Accountability measures are quality measures designed to produce the greatest positive impact on the outcomes of individuals receiving care when health care organizations demonstrate improvement in a given process. The Joint Commission categorizes measures into two categories: accountability and non-accountability measures. Measures that meet established criteria should be used for purposes of accountability (for example, accreditation, public reporting, or pay-for-performance). Alternately, measures that have not been designated as accountability measures may be useful for PI and learning within individual health care organizations.

TOOL

Measurement Evaluation Checklist

Process Measures

In the last two decades, a plethora of new process measures has arisen. The good news is that many of them are good measures that meet these criteria. That is, they measure whether well-applied, proven clinical practices are improving outcomes for individuals receiving care, adjusting for the effects of other procedures and differences in the population(s) of individuals served, and do not incentivize bad or unhelpful behaviors. But you must be careful and vigilant when designing or adopting new measures to ensure that they meet the following stringent criteria:

- **Research.** Strong scientific evidence demonstrates that performing the evidence-based process improves health outcomes—either directly or by reducing the risk of adverse outcomes.
- **Proximity.** Performing the care process is closely connected to the care recipient outcome; there are relatively few clinical processes that occur after the one that is measured and before the improved outcome occurs.
- **Accuracy.** The measure accurately assesses whether or not the care process has actually been provided. That is, the measure should be capable of indicating whether the process has been delivered with sufficient effectiveness to make improved outcomes likely.
- **Adverse effects.** Implementing the measure has little or no chance of inducing unintended adverse consequences.

Outcome Measures

Outcome measures are metrics that indicate the result of performance (or nonperformance) of a function(s) or process(es). An outcome measure should be used only if the outcome can be influenced substantially by providers (for example, if a strong process–outcome link exists, and differences in outcomes are truly attributable to differences in the care provided; that is, statistical adjustment can be made for differences in care recipient populations across providers).* To evaluate accountability outcome measures for your organization, use the following criteria:

- **Evidence.** Strong evidence should exist that good medical care leads to improvement in the outcome within the time period for the measure.
- **Precision.** The outcome should be measurable with a high degree of precision.
- **Risk adjustment.** The risk-adjustment methodology should include and accurately measure the risk factors most strongly associated with the outcomes.
- **Minimal adverse effects.** Implementation of the outcome measure must have little chance of causing adverse consequences.

Although many of the measures you will use to collect and report your PI data will be standardized measures developed by The Joint Commission and/or regulatory agencies, these criteria should guide your thinking should you decide to design your own PI measures and projects.

---

* Baker DW, Chassin MR. Holding providers accountable for health care outcomes. *Ann Intern Med.* 2017 Sep 19;167(6):418–423.

WHY DO I NEED TO KNOW THIS NOW?

Familiarity with quality measures and the methodology behind their development will help you understand the reporting requirements and evaluate new tools and measures as you encounter them. Many of the existing process and outcome measures are good measures that meet accountability criteria. That is, they measure whether well-applied, proven, evidence-based clinical practices are improving outcomes for individuals receiving care, and they do not incentivize bad or unhelpful behaviors. However, you must be careful and vigilant when designing or adopting new measures to ensure that they meet the stringent criteria listed for process and outcome accountability measures.

WHERE DO I START?

- **Learn more.** If applicable to your organization, familiarize yourself with ORYX® performance measures. ORYX performance measures integrate a variety of evidence-based measures for use in the assisted living community, hospital, and critical access hospital accreditation process and are therefore a valuable source of high-quality measures.

"I heard that...

there's no such thing as 'good enough' on performance measures. Organizations should strive for 100% performance."

fact:

The goal may not be 100% for some measures. No measure can possibly address every potential clinical scenario. Through the evaluation of best practice and clinical judgment, caregivers provide high-quality care and continue to identify opportunities for improvement. Measurement supports continuous quality improvement.

KEY CONCEPT

ORYX® MEASURES

The Joint Commission has a primary focus on adopting accountability measures for its ORYX® program:

- The Joint Commission's ORYX initiative integrates performance measurement data into the accreditation process.
- ORYX measurement requirements support Joint Commission-accredited organizations in their quality improvement efforts.
- The Joint Commission continues to align measures as closely as possible with the Centers for Medicare & Medicaid Services (CMS).

The Joint Commission will continue to reexamine all process (that is, proportion and ratio) measures categorized as accountability measures to ensure that they continue to meet the accountability criteria. Organizations are encouraged to keep up to date on any changes in the ORYX requirements by reviewing recent issues of *Perspectives* or by going to the "Measurement" area on The Joint Commission's website.

Specifications Manuals

Available on The Joint Commission's website, Electronic Clinical Quality Measures and Chart Abstracted Measures contain specific information about each of the quality measures The Joint Commission uses as part of its ORYX reporting requirements for accreditation, including all the data elements required for each. In addition, the Electronic Clinical Quality Improvement (eCQI) Resource Center provides electronic clinical quality measures (eCQMs) information that is used by both The Joint Commission and CMS.

(See "Recommended Resources" near the end of this book for links to the manuals and the eCQI Resource Center.)

WHY DO I NEED TO KNOW THIS NOW?

If you are an accreditation professional working in a health care organization with reporting requirements, you need to be informed about ORYX and know what data need to be reported to The Joint Commission.

WHERE DO I START?

- **Educate yourself about performance measurement and its requirements.** Know what requirements your organization must comply with to sustain accreditation. Visit The Joint Commission's "Measurement" webpage to learn more about performance measurement and ORYX specifically.
- **Meet with quality control staff.** As you meet and begin working with various staff throughout your organization, make sure to connect with any quality department staff or other staff members who are responsible for gathering performance measurement data.
- **Review the specifications manuals.** The Joint Commission updates its eCQM specification manual annually and its chart-abstracted specifications manual semiannually. Make sure to familiarize yourself with these manuals and note any changes to reporting requirements that affect your organization.

TOOL

eCQM Systems and Processes Update Procedure Checklist

Test Your Knowledge

1. State whether each of the following is a process, an outcome, or a continuous variable performance measure:
   a. Percentage of patients receiving pneumococcal vaccination
   b. Hand hygiene compliance
   c. Surgical site infection rate for orthopedic procedures
   d. Number of emergency department visits for asthma
   e. Clinic wait time
   f. Clinical guidelines applied for patients with severe sepsis
   g. Readmission within 30 days

2. An organization had a readmission rate that was the lowest in the region. As a result, the Centers for Medicare & Medicaid Services reimbursed the organization an extra percent. Which of the following would best describe this type of measure?
   - ☐ a. Performance
   - ☐ b. Leapfrog
   - ☐ c. 5 star
   - ☐ d. Accountability

3. Which of the following statements are true about The Joint Commission's performance measurement program for hospitals? (Select all that apply.)
   - ☐ a. The name of the program is ORYX®.
   - ☐ b. The Joint Commission works with the Centers for Medicare & Medicaid Services for alignment of measurements.
   - ☐ c. All of the measures are electronically extracted from the EHR.
   - ☐ d. The program is voluntary for accredited hospitals.

CHAPTER 8

Working with Data

THE BIG IDEA

As part of maintaining your accreditation, certification, verification, and, if applicable, other quality reporting programs, you will need to collect and report data on the performance of your organization. In this chapter we will cover important points about data collection and identify the major entities to which you may have to report those data.

KEY CONCEPTS

- Collecting Data
- Reporting Data
- Displaying Data
- Putting the Data to Work

THE MANUAL

Following are the relevant Joint Commission E-dition® or *Comprehensive Accreditation Manual* chapters:

- "Accreditation Participation Requirements" (APR)
- "Information Management" (IM)
- "Performance Improvement" (PI)
- "Performance Measurement and the ORYX Initiative" (PM) [assisted living community, critical access hospital, and hospital only]

PRIORITY

Using Data to Improve Health Care Equity

Our vision at The Joint Commission is that all people always experience safe, high-quality health care. Today, however, health care quality and health outcomes are often worse for racial/ethnic minorities, women, people living in rural communities, people with disabilities, those living in poverty, people with lower educational attainment, and other historically marginalized groups.

Although health care equity is often viewed through a social justice lens, we at The Joint Commission understand it to be first and foremost a quality-of-care problem. This means to achieve sustainable improvement we need to approach health care equity in the same way we approach other crucial patient safety priorities—by understanding the root causes and implementing targeted standards of care.

State-of-the-art health care equity accreditation standards, which are now a National Patient Safety Goal, help organizations put patients at the heart of everything they do. One of the steps toward health equity is collecting data on the patient's health-related social needs as part of this National Patient Safety Goal. The Health Care Equity Resource Center on The Joint Commission's website can help your organization get started. Working side by side, we can write a new chapter.

KEY CONCEPT

COLLECTING DATA

Even though innovations in information technology have made the collection and aggregation of data much more efficient in recent years, the task of collecting meaningful performance data can still be time consuming and daunting. The following are some guidelines to follow as you address this critical task in both the accreditation process and your own performance improvement (PI) program.

Valid and Reliable Information

Improving the quality of care, treatment, and services and the reliability of your organization is only possible through focused PI activities. These activities, in turn, rely on the collection of valid and reliable data about current performance. As explained in Chapter 7, you cannot overestimate the importance of evidence-based measures. These measures must then be applied consistently and carefully, including monitoring to ensure that the measures themselves are not creating unintended adverse outcomes. The usefulness of the information and analysis you gain will be directly proportional to the care you take to ensure that data are collected accurately and that they precisely measure the process or outcome you want them to.

Standardized Data Collection

Toward the goal of ensuring accuracy and reliability of data, you should institute one or more methods for how the data are collected and recorded. You can't meaningfully compare apples to oranges, after all. Think about who will be collecting the data and how, using what methods and technology. Then try to think of ways to make it easier for collectors or recorders of data to do so in a consistent and standardized way. What units will be used? What data elements will be required?

Data Integrity

Just as the validity of your data is critical to their being useful, the integrity of the data must also be ensured. This means that your data must be collected, stored, and transmitted securely. Any changes to the data must be documented, and the history of such changes must be secure from alteration or deletion. Regular backups, as in any other information management system, are highly recommended to prevent data loss or theft.

Method of Collection

Outside of regular PI projects, in which data may be collected through interviews and direct observation, you will often be required to amass large data sets. There are two main methods of large-scale data collection.

- **Chart-abstracted collection.** In this method data collectors will review records of care and other sources to collect the needed data.

- **Electronic clinical quality measures (eCQMs).** As the health care industry has increasingly moved away from paper records and toward electronic recordkeeping, most performance measure data are being collected from electronic health records (EHRs) and other digital sources. Organizations submitting electronic data to The Joint Commission use the Quality Reporting Document Architecture (QRDA), which is a standard document format for the exchange of eCQM data. The QRDA creates a standard method to exchange eCQM data between systems. The QRDA file may be created by the organization or with the assistance of an EHR vendor or quality reporting vendor that is contracted to create the needed files for reporting. The same version of the QRDA file is used for submission to The Joint Commission and other regulatory agencies (such as the US Centers for Medicare & Medicaid Services [CMS]).

WHY DO I NEED TO KNOW THIS NOW?

Data collection is a foundation of PI in any segment of health care. Many accredited organizations or those seeking accreditation also now need to collect data on care recipients' health-related social needs (HRSNs) as part of the National Patient Safety Goal on health care equity. The key is to identify and collect meaningful data that can have a positive influence on your organization's performance. You can't start doing this "sometime soon." It must be now, and it must be ongoing. Knowing what data are collected, where they come from, how they are consistently collected, what they are used for, and when they are available will help you establish strategies for managing those data.

WHERE DO I START?

- **Organize information.** Identify internal and external sources of data to start. Then work with your team, perhaps with help from the information technology team, health records team, and quality team, to improve your data collection efforts by creating a standardized database and keeping it updated.
- **Collaborate with experts.** Work with PI experts in your organization (or a PI consultant) to ensure that you are identifying and collecting meaningful data.
- **Consult resources.** Check E-dition or your *Comprehensive Accreditation Manual* to make sure you are familiar with the PI standards, as well as the standards that require documentation. Documentation may include data collection.

KEY CONCEPT

REPORTING DATA

Where do all those data go? Well, there are several destinations and routes. You will be required to submit specific performance data to The Joint Commission for the purposes of meeting accreditation, certification, and/or verification participation requirements. Also, there may be external agencies, including government entities, to which you may want or be required to report these data.

Direct Data Submission Platform (DDSP)

Joint Commission–accredited health care organizations have access to the DDSP for submission of eCQM and chart-abstracted data. The DDSP allows accredited organizations to directly submit eCQM and chart-abstracted data to The Joint Commission to reduce reporting burden and expense and to empower organizations with valid data for measurement and analysis in ongoing health care quality improvement. Key benefits of the DDSP include the following:

- 24-hour-a-day/7-day-a-week access during the submission period
- Easy-to-use data visuals
- Cloud-based platform environment with fast file transfer
- State-of-the-art rules engine
- Transparency

Certification Measure Information Process (CMIP)

The Joint Commission integrates the receipt of performance measurement data into the certification process. The Certification Measure Information Process (CMIP) tool is applicable to all health care organizations that are currently certified or are seeking certification for the first time. The CMIP tool has an electronic form that hospitals use to submit certification performance measurement data and performance improvement information to The Joint Commission.

For any questions related to the Certification process, please contact your account executive.

Information on how and when to submit these data is available on your *Joint Commission Connect®* extranet site.

External Quality Data Reporting

You may be required or choose to report performance data to several governmental and public health agencies or programs. These may include but are not limited to the following:

- US Centers for Disease Control and Prevention (CDC)
    - National Healthcare Safety Network (NHSN)
- US Centers for Medicare & Medicaid Services (CMS) Quality Reporting Programs
    - Hospital Inpatient Quality Reporting Program (HIQR)
    - Hospital Outpatient Quality Reporting Program (HOQR)
    - Promoting Interoperability Programs
    - Inpatient Psychiatric Facility Quality Reporting Program (IPFQR)
    - Inpatient Rehabilitation Facilities (IRF)
    - Long-Term Care Hospital Quality Reporting Program (LTCH QRP)
    - Ambulatory Surgical Center Quality Reporting Program (ASCQR)
    - Home Health Quality Reporting Program (HH QRP)
    - Skilled Nursing Facility Quality Reporting Program (SNF QRP)

WHY DO I NEED TO KNOW THIS NOW?

If you can collect and assess meaningful performance data, you can make better decisions about your own current performance and the results of PI projects. Also, you will need to report certain data to The Joint Commission and assorted governmental agencies.

WHERE DO I START?

- **Review requirements.** The specifications manuals for measure reporting on The Joint Commission's website will guide you through Joint Commission– and CMS–required data reporting. For other health care settings, familiarize yourself with any other data reporting required by law and regulation.
- **Create a reporting calendar.** It will probably be helpful to create a reporting calendar to keep track of what data need to be collected and submitted when.
- **Measure continuously.** To fuel continuous improvement, you need continuous monitoring and measuring.

KEY CONCEPT

DISPLAYING DATA

All those data you are collecting aren't just for reporting to The Joint Commission and regulatory agencies used for deemed status. They can be useful to you and to the public at large. Presenting data in visual formats, such as graphs, charts, flowcharts, and diagrams, can be invaluable in helping managers and leaders understand difficult concepts suggested by the data or just to see trends in a way that may be more difficult when reading raw numbers.

Benchmarking

Data can be used to establish performance benchmarks and comparison groups. Data aggregated across the industry or sector or geographic area can be used to give organizational leaders a sense of how they are doing and what appropriate PI targets might look like or where to focus specific efforts for improvement.

Accelerate PI™

The Joint Commission has created a series of dashboards for selected accredited organizations that have available standardized performance measures. The dashboards are available to Joint Commission–accredited ambulatory surgery centers, home health and hospice organizations, hospitals, critical access hospitals, long-term care hospitals, inpatient psychiatric facilities, inpatient rehabilitation facilities, and nursing care centers. These dashboards present performance data visually by using publicly available data sets from CMS. The dashboards, titled Accelerate PI, are available on your *Joint Commission Connect* extranet site. The dashboard notes each organization's performance on selected measures. For each measure, the dashboard shows that organization's performance compared to national, state, and Joint Commission–accredited organization averages. Joint Commission surveyors are trained to use the dashboards to frame survey discussions on quality improvement priorities and activities. The dashboard is not a scorable element on survey but a tool to facilitate discussion about ongoing quality improvement. The dashboards contain information on vetted, reliable, quality measures, as well as various helpful benchmarks and direct links to topic-specific quality improvement resources.

WHY DO I NEED TO KNOW THIS NOW?

Data reporting serves the purpose of stimulating continuous improvement at every level, from the unit level to the organization level to the industry level, with the goal of zero harm. Benchmarking and data visualizations such as dashboards give a starting point to the conversation and highlight opportunities for improvement.

WHERE DO I START?

- **Learn more.** A substantial part of the job of an accreditation professional is the collection, analysis, and use of data to help maintain compliance and improve performance. Although The Joint Commission and other entities will aggregate, analyze, and present data for you in ways that may inform your PI activities and help you better maintain compliance, it's critical for you to understand data gathering and statistical analysis methods yourself so that you can apply them in your PI program.

PICTURE THIS

Seeing Your Performance Improvement

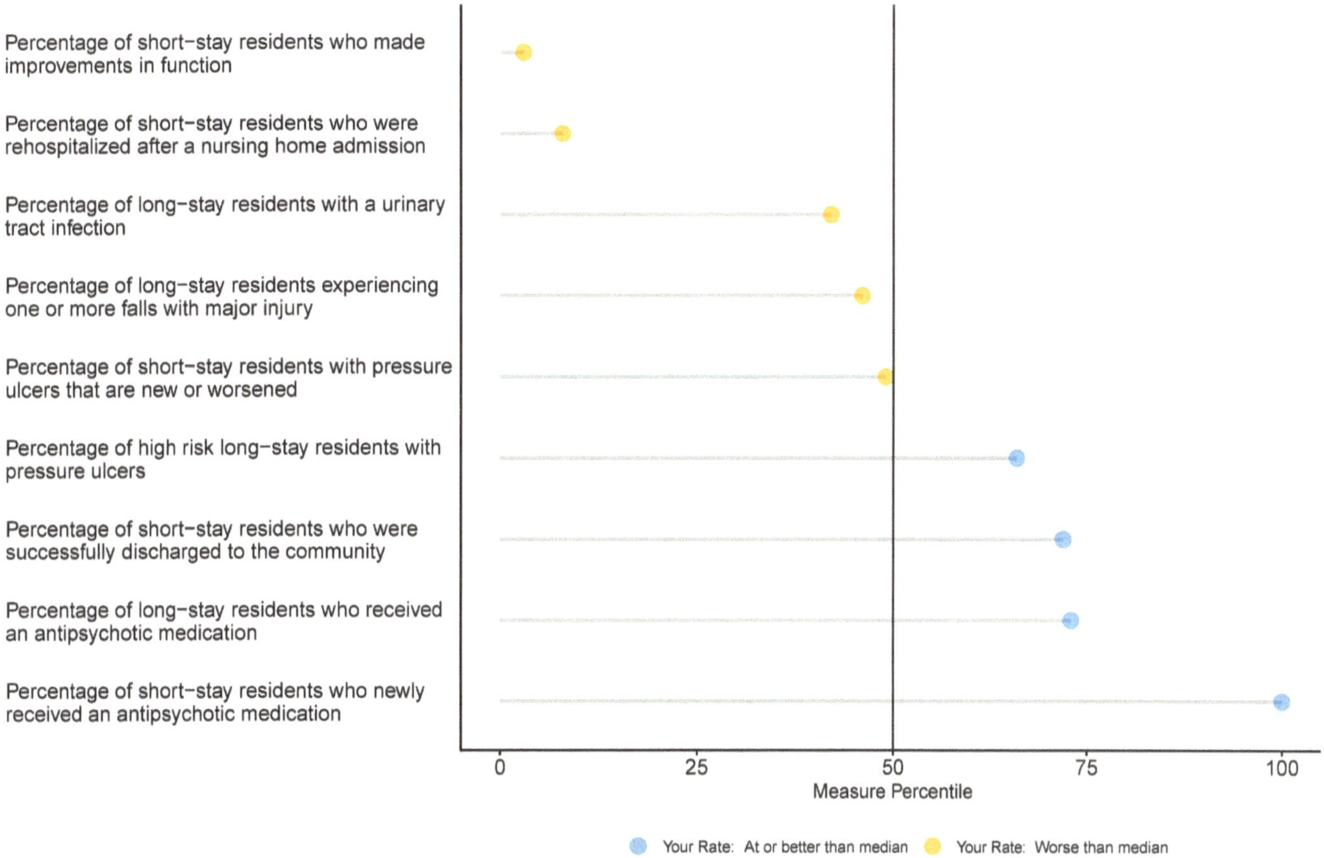

The Joint Commission launched Accelerate PI to provide performance measurement data on select measures. This report is intended to be a springboard for conversations on data, performance measures, and quality improvement during the survey process. In addition, the report is a valuable ongoing resource for accredited organizations.

KEY CONCEPT

PUTTING THE DATA TO WORK

Accreditation and PI professionals can present information about organizational performance to leaders in a way that allows leaders to understand what the organization is doing well and what it can improve upon, relative to peer organizations and the health care industry. Leaders can then use this information to inform decisions about PI and other safety improvement activities.

Using Collected Data as a Prioritization Tool

Data collected as part of mandatory reporting, as well as data collected as part of normal PI activities, are invaluable tools for spotting big or long-term trends in performance and operations. These trends can help inform leaders' decisions about the long-term strategy and direction of the organization.

Tools to Identify Trends

There is no shortage of data available to review and analyze organizational performance. In addition to the data your organization collects, look at other recent data sources to identify performance trends that require follow-up improvement activities.

Mock tracers. Review mock tracers that have recently been conducted. What issues were recorded? Do you have data that support or refute findings from the mock tracer?

***Survey Analysis for Evaluating Risk*® (*SAFER*®) Matrix data.** You can use *SAFER* data collected during a mock tracer or review the biannually published top noncompliance standards to determine where and if trends appear.

TOOL

Data Analysis Procedure Checklist

Accelerate PI. These dashboards provide valuable information that may help you determine what PI activities need to be addressed and how soon they need to be addressed.

WHY DO I NEED TO KNOW THIS NOW?

Making the right decisions about when and how to change how care, treatment, and services are delivered or about the long-term course of the organization requires meaningful data to be collected, analyzed, and presented to those with the power to make change. Poorly designed measures, errors or inconsistencies, data gaps, and suboptimal presentation may lead to poor decision-making or delays in recognizing important trends.

WHERE DO I START?

- **Encourage technology use.** The more health care data are recorded in digital formats, the easier it is to collect, organize, and analyze them.
- **Facilitate processes.** Beware of interoperability problems and differing standards in recording information. Ensure that your various information management systems can talk to one another and that as many of the data fields as possible are standardized across platforms. It's a challenge, but it can make using these systems and extracting meaningful data from them much easier.
- **Link to PI resources.** Joint Commission standards require each accredited organization to conduct PI activities. These activities are meant to help organizations identify areas for improvement and plan improvement actions identified either by the PI activities or on survey. When data are collected, analyzed, and presented in an accurate and compelling format, and compared to well-established benchmarks, they can be meaningful and helpful in informing organizational decisions.

TOOL

Proposed Performance Improvement Project Decision Checklist

Test Your Knowledge

1. Which of the following is the data submission platform for Joint Commission certification programs?
   - ☐ a. Electronic Clinical Quality Measures (eCQM)
   - ☐ b. Certification Measure Information Process (CMIP)
   - ☐ c. Centers for Medicare & Medicaid Services (CMS)
   - ☐ d. International Organization for Standardization (ISO) Certification

2. The Direct Data Submission Platform (DDSP) ___. (Select all that apply.)
   - ☐ a. can receive data only from approved data warehouse vendors
   - ☐ b. is available during normal business hours
   - ☐ c. can receive chart-abstracted data
   - ☐ d. can receive Quality Reporting Document Architecture (QRDA)

3. Based on the chapter, which of the following best describes the process sequence for working with data?
   - ☐ a. Reporting, collecting, displaying, putting the data to work
   - ☐ b. Collecting, displaying, putting the data to work, reporting
   - ☐ c. Collecting, reporting, displaying, putting the data to work
   - ☐ d. Putting the data to work, displaying, reporting, collecting

4. Which of the following can adversely affect the output of your data analysis process? (Select all that apply.)
   - ☐ a. Inconsistent data definitions
   - ☐ b. Different individuals collecting data
   - ☐ c. Lack of data validation
   - ☐ d. Current specification manual

PART 4
Understanding Challenging Standards

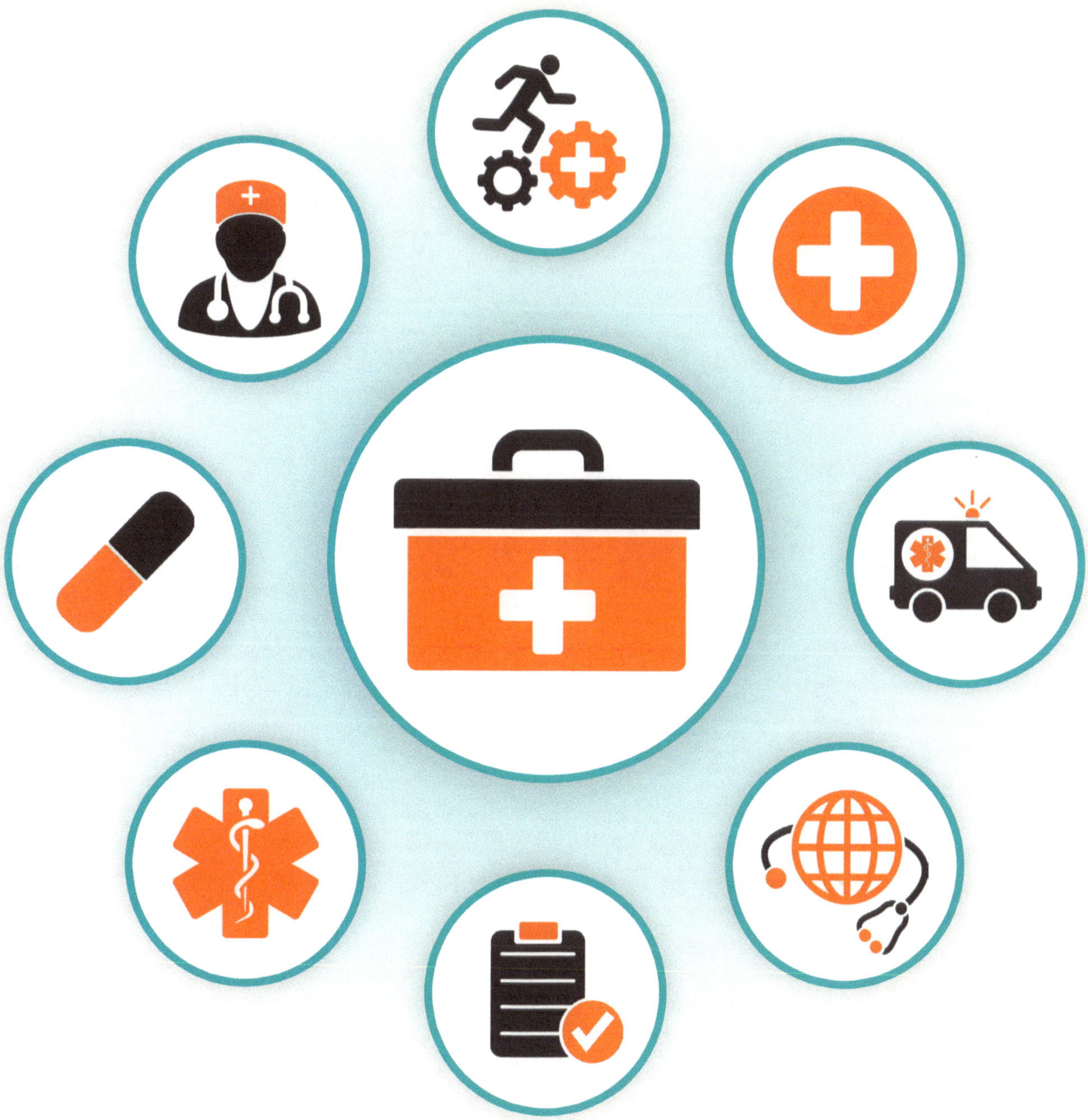

Part 4 is an overview of Joint Commission standards. Readers should always go to E-edition® or their *Comprehensive Accreditation Manual* to get the most up-to-date requirements to follow. The standards are listed alphabetically, as they are in the manuals and on E-dition.

Care, Treatment, and Services

CHAPTER 9

THE BIG IDEA

Care, treatment, and services for care recipients depend on a safe and effective customized delivery system, which is made up of many processes. It must be well designed and organized and consistently and appropriately implemented. The process crosses all departments, service lines, and settings. It involves planning, assessing, providing, and coordinating of all care, treatment, and services, as well as ensuring the safety of the care recipient and others. Throughout the process, providers, staff, and care recipients communicate openly about the rights as well as the responsibilities of the care recipient as a member of the care delivery team.

KEY CONCEPTS

- Planning and Coordinating Care, Treatment, and Services
- Assessment and Reassessment
- Restraint and Seclusion
- Operative or High-Risk Procedures
- Safety Risks
- Rights and Responsibilities of Care Recipients

THE MANUAL

Following are the relevant Joint Commission E-dition® or *Comprehensive Accreditation Manual* chapters:

- "Care, Treatment, and Services" (CTS) [behavioral health care and human services only]
- "Medication Management" (MM) [not laboratory]
- "National Patient Safety Goals" (NPSG)
- "Provision of Care, Treatment, and Services" (PC) [not behavioral health care and human services or laboratory]
- "Rights and Responsibilities of the Individual" (RI) [not laboratory]

Top Challenging Care, Treatment, and Services Standards

The following standards and elements of performance (EPs) are those which have recently been most frequently cited by surveyors as being non-compliant.

Standard	Element of Performance (EP)	Applicable Accreditation Program(s)
PC.01.03.01: The organization plans the patient's care.	**EP 5:** The written plan of care is based on the patient's goals and the time frames, settings, and services required to meet those goals.	Home Care
PC.01.03.01: The organization plans the patient's care.	**EP 10:** For home health agencies that elect to use The Joint Commission deemed status option: The individualized plan of care specifies the care and services necessary to meet the needs identified in the comprehensive assessment and addresses the following: • All pertinent diagnoses • Mental, psychosocial, and cognitive status • Types of services, supplies, and equipment required • The frequency and duration of visits • The patient's prognosis • The patient's potential for rehabilitation • The patient's functional limitations • The patient's permitted activities • The patient's nutritional requirements • All medications and treatments • Safety measures to protect against injury • A description of the patient's risk for emergency department visits and hospital readmission, and all necessary interventions to address the underlying risk factors • Patient-specific interventions and education • Measurable outcomes and goals identified by the organization and patient as a result of implementing and coordinating the plan of care • Patient and caregiver education and training to facilitate timely discharge • Information related to any advance directives • Identification of the disciplines involved in providing care • Any other relevant items, including additions, revisions, and deletions that the home health agency, physician, or allowed practitioner may choose to include	Home Care
PC.01.03.01: The organization plans the patient's care.	**EP 18:** For hospices that elect to use The Joint Commission deemed status option: The plan of care includes all services needed for the palliation and management of the terminal illness and related conditions, including the following: • Interventions to manage pain and symptoms • A statement of the scope and frequency of the services necessary to meet the patient's and family's needs • Measurable outcomes anticipated from implementing and coordinating the plan of care • Medications and treatment necessary to meet the patient's needs • Medical supplies and appliances necessary to meet the patient's needs	Home Care

Standard	EP	Applicable Accreditation Program(s)
PC.01.03.01: The organization plans the patient's care.	**EP 55:** For home health agencies that elect to use The Joint Commission deemed status option: There is a plan for the patient that provides instructions if there is an emergency in the organization or the community that might disrupt the care, treatment, or service provided by the organization. This plan is based on the patient's assessed needs, including clinical, functional, and communication needs; reliance upon equipment or assistive devices; and available caregiver support.	Home Care
PC.02.01.03: The organization provides care, treatment, or services in accordance with orders or prescriptions, as required by law and regulation.	**EP 1:** Prior to providing care, the organization obtains or renews orders (verbal or written) from a physician or allowed practitioner in accordance with professional standards of practice and law and regulation.	Home Care
PC.02.01.11: Resuscitative services are available throughout the hospital.	**EP 2:** Resuscitation equipment is available for use based on the needs of the population served.	Hospital

PICTURE THIS

Interdisciplinary Care Planning

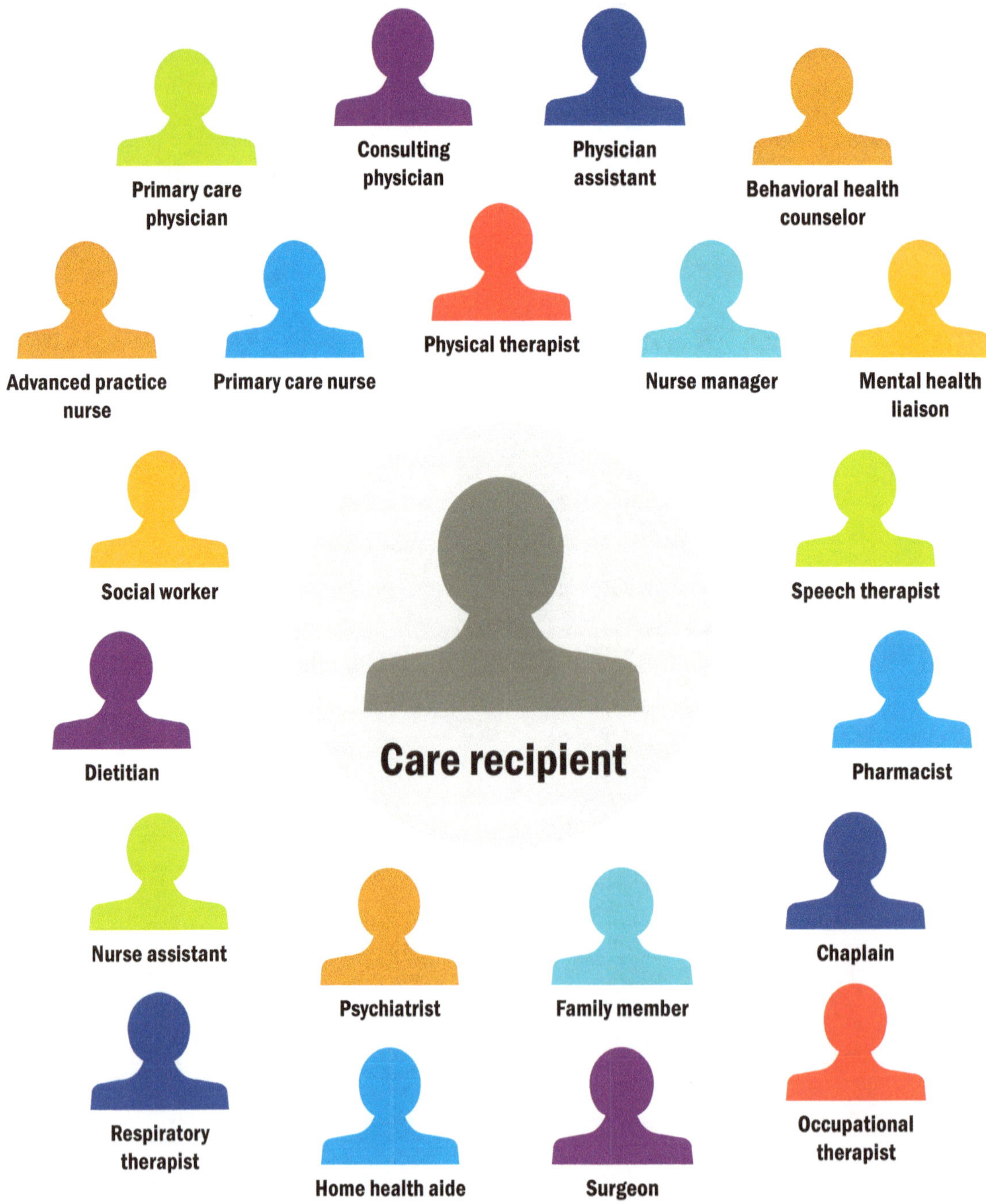

Few care recipients are only under the care of nurses and physicians. Any of the above caregivers could be engaged in the plan of care, ideally as part of an interdisciplinary team. An interdisciplinary approach to care—one that draws on a wide spectrum of knowledge, experience, and expertise—is proven to improve the health care experience for care recipients, providers, and health care organizations alike.

KEY CONCEPT

PLANNING AND COORDINATING CARE, TREATMENT, AND SERVICES

All needs, always: Care planning should reflect all of a care recipient's needs at any point in the care process. The emphasis should always be on individualized care plans derived from the individual's history and physical as well as input from family and nursing assessments, as applicable. Effective care plans are flexible, realistic, simple, useful, informative, individualized, care recipient–centered, supportive, and collaborative.

TOOL

Interdisciplinary Care Plan Evaluation Checklist

Coordination of Care

The Joint Commission standards require an interdisciplinary, collaborative approach to coordination of care. This interdisciplinary approach should have specific goals and time frames established to meet those goals. This can be accomplished best with an interdisciplinary team of caregivers that includes the care recipient whenever possible. The team works together, creating and adjusting the care plan, evaluating progress toward goals, engaging in interventions based on the care plan, updating the electronic health record (EHR),* and keeping everyone informed. That kind of teamwork remains important during continuing care and any transition of care to ensure continuity when the care recipient is referred, transferred, or discharged.

Discharge Planning

Although the long-term goal of any transition of care is to ensure continuity, the immediate goal of discharge planning is to anticipate changes in individual care needs. After discharge (known as the "end of an episode of care" in some settings), a health care team's oversight of a care recipient becomes more limited. For that reason, the care recipient and family need to be involved in discharge planning. The Joint Commission requires care recipient/family education at discharge as well. Are the care recipient's medication orders clear to the individual? Does the care recipient know what symptoms to watch out for? Does the family have any questions? Who will be following up with the care recipient after discharge?

TOOL

Discharge Summary Evaluation Checklist

WHY DO I NEED TO KNOW THIS NOW?

Knowing the proven effectiveness of interdisciplinary care planning will give you the confidence to encourage this approach in your organization—not only to meet the requirements but to support safety and quality for all care recipients.

---

* The Joint Commission does not require health records to be electronic.

PICTURE THIS

Effective Care Plans

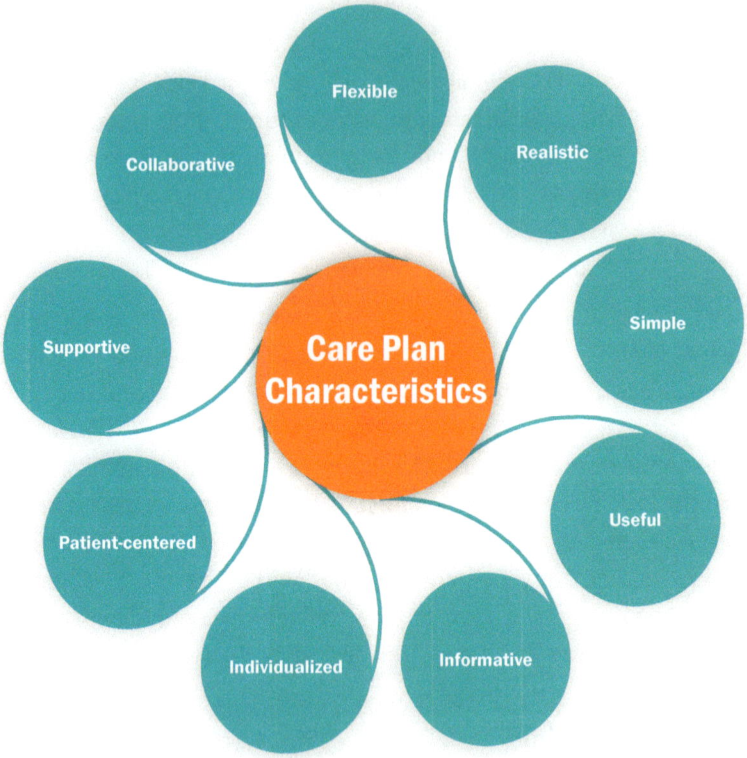

"I heard that...

care plans can be standardized."

fact

Every care recipient is a unique combination of symptoms, history, behaviors, physiology, and so on. It only makes sense that every care recipient deserves a comprehensive, customized care plan. On the other hand, you can standardize a format for a care plan, which may help to ensure that all aspects of every care recipient's care are always addressed.

WHERE DO I START?

- **Learn more.** Familiarize yourself with the PC standards (CTS for behavioral health care and human services) and the NPSG requirements applicable to your population(s). Go through them one by one and record your comments, concerns, and questions. Then follow up by talking to your colleagues or The Joint Commission for further clarification, as needed.
- **Review documents.** Review your organization's policies covering care planning, assessment, coordination of care, and discharge planning. See any need for improvements? Call together an interdisciplinary review team and ask for input.
- **Encourage technology use.** If you're using an EHR system, think about incorporating electronic interdisciplinary care plans that clinicians on the care team can access from any computer. Information in the EHR populates the plan-of-care screen.
- **Facilitate processes.** Discharge summaries are required to facilitate transitions of care. Ask staff to use a checklist so you're sure each discharge summary includes all the necessary elements and is properly delivered. The Joint Commission does not require a checklist, but it could be used as a best practice in your organization.

KEY CONCEPT

ASSESSMENT AND REASSESSMENT

All care planning includes assessment and reassessment. An assessment must be conducted whenever there's a change in the care recipient's condition and/or within certain time frames (determined by your organization's policy and law and regulation). The initial assessment often includes a nutritional and functional screening.

Specialized Assessment and Reassessment Processes

Certain health conditions require specialized assessment and reassessment processes. Some of these are more common in certain health care settings.

- **Pressure ulcers.** This is vital for assisted living communities, nursing care centers, and home care organizations, where care recipients may spend long periods in bed. Daily checks can significantly decrease or eliminate pressure ulcers.
- **Suicide risk.** In non–behavioral health care and human services settings, staff may need training in suicide risk screening and assessment. You'll also need to establish a process for monitoring at-risk care recipients and documenting monitoring efforts.
- **Falls.** This is a top priority in many settings. Programs targeting falls risk are common in hospitals, critical access hospitals, assisted living communities, nursing care centers, and home care.

WHY DO I NEED TO KNOW THIS NOW?

Assessment and reassessment are part of the foundational circle of health care. As an accreditation professional, this is an area to watch closely, as many standards relate to it.

WHERE DO I START?

- **Review documents.** Pull together members of a current care recipient's interdisciplinary care team in your organization. Does the plan of care used for that individual conform to your organization's policies and procedures? Do your policies and procedures reflect Joint Commission requirements?
- **Conduct tracers.** Perform periodic, targeted mini-tracers to be sure staff are following policies for reassessment. Look for the following:
  - Awareness of what reassessments are necessary
  - Recognition of where and how to document assessments and reassessments
  - Ability to assess and reassess care recipients who are nonverbal or not oriented (including any infant and pediatric care recipients)
- **Provide training.** Help staff get any necessary training for suicide risk screening and assessment. Make sure they use a standardized form and process for documentation and response. Note that a screening would be the

initial review of the care recipient's suicidality. A suicide assessment would be significantly more detailed and conducted by a trained professional, resulting in determining a level of suicide risk. These two activities are very different and should not be considered as interchangeable. See "Recommended Resources" for free online resources you can use.

PICTURE THIS

Circle of Health Care Assessment and Reassessment

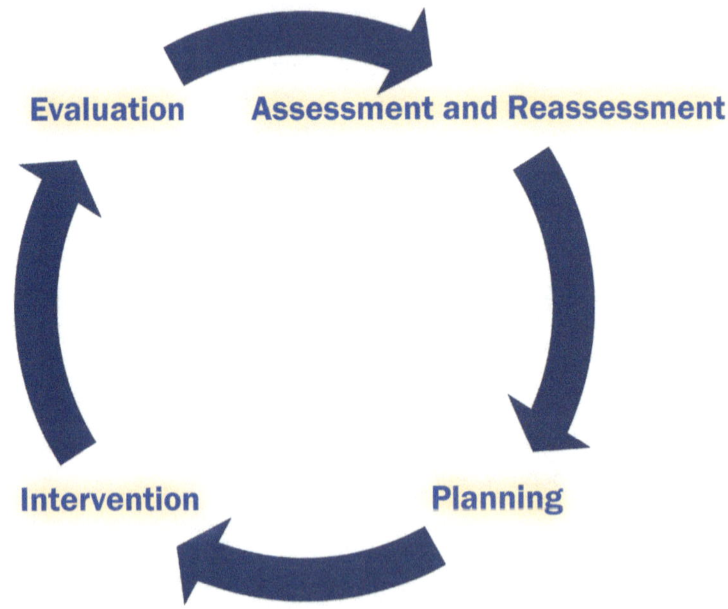

The foundational circle of health care includes the four phases of assessment, planning, intervention, and evaluation. The same pattern repeats itself with every care interaction, and it all begins with assessment or reassessment.

KEY CONCEPT

RESTRAINT AND SECLUSION

Restraint and seclusion are sensitive subjects for health care professionals. Misuse of restraint and seclusion can cause psychological harm, violate the care recipient's rights, and result in serious injury and/or death. Certainly, specific situations do occur in which restraining or secluding a care recipient has legitimate clinical or emergency behavioral value. Overall, however, these methods should be carefully assessed and monitored at the organizational level to avoid unnecessary or inappropriate use and to ensure regulatory compliance.

Restraint for Medical Reasons

Restraints are allowable when standard practices deem them clinically appropriate to a care recipient's medical care. A few examples are intravenous arm boards, orthopedic appliances, protective helmets, and restraints used during surgical procedures. Individual orders should be given for these cases.

Restraint for Security and Behavioral Health Reasons

In certain emergency situations, safety demands a physical response. The goal is to prevent those circumstances from developing in the first place. Care recipients with emotional or behavioral disorders may need to be restrained or secluded to keep them from injuring themselves or others. Nonphysical methods should be used whenever possible. Restraining an individual may also occur when required by law enforcement for security reasons.

General Criteria for Restraint

If restraint or seclusion is necessary, its approved use should meet these general criteria:

- Based on care recipient needs
- Order-driven
- Adhered to the organization's written policies and procedures
- Time limited
- Reevaluated frequently by qualified staff
- Discontinued as soon as possible

WHY DO I NEED TO KNOW THIS NOW?

It's crucial for you to know what's appropriate and when in order to help prevent incidents and to address compliance issues. You can't afford to say, "I didn't know."

WHERE DO I START?

- **Learn more.** The Joint Commission has many standards addressing restraint and seclusion. Familiarize yourself with the acceptable uses of restraint as defined in the standards. Know your organization's status (deemed or not) to be sure you're following the right protocols. Then examine your organization's relevant policies and procedures, looking for guidelines that answer these questions:
    - When is restraint or seclusion considered?
    - Who can initiate the use of restraint or seclusion?
    - How often is a care recipient in restraint or seclusion to be evaluated/reevaluated?
    - Who can reevaluate a care recipient in restraint or seclusion?
    - If a care recipient is in restraint or seclusion, is an order required within a short time after initiation?
    - Is an order required to identify and initiate a need for restraint or seclusion?
    - How often do orders for the use of restraint or seclusion need to be renewed?

KEY CONCEPT

OPERATIVE OR HIGH-RISK PROCEDURES

Good communication, teamwork, care recipient involvement, complementary strategies, consistent implementation of standardized protocols: Those are principles integral to nearly any safe care, treatment, or services of care recipients. They're critical ones for operative or high-risk procedures. That's when care recipients often feel, and sometimes are, the most vulnerable.

Preanesthesia Evaluation

The risk is greatest for care recipients who require moderate to deep sedation or anesthesia. An individual under moderate or deep sedation loses protective reflexes. A care recipient under anesthesia can't be roused or respond in any fashion. Under the PC standards, the organization must perform a preanesthesia evaluation for the care recipient. This can be part of the preprocedural visit, but it serves a distinct purpose.

For deemed status. You must meet specific requirements for who's qualified to perform the preanesthesia and postanesthesia evaluations and timing of those evaluations. However, organizations do have some flexibility in the format and process for the evaluations.

The Universal Protocol

Wrong. Wrong. Wrong. Performing the wrong procedure, on the wrong care recipient, or at the wrong site can and must be prevented. The Universal Protocol for Preventing Wrong Site, Wrong Procedure, and Wrong Person Surgery™ is designed to do just that by application of these three components:

- **Conducting a preprocedure verification process.** Making sure the right procedure will be performed on the right care recipient happens first. All relevant documents and equipment should be available and matched to the care recipient. Involving the care recipient whenever possible is required.
- **Marking the procedure site.** This is a must whenever there's more than one possible location for a procedure—limbs, lesions, level of the spine, and so on. A consistent, clearly understood marking process used throughout your organization works best. Involving the care recipient if possible is required at this point too.
- **Performing a time-out.** Just before the procedure begins, the whole team stops everything and actively confirms the correct care recipient, procedure, and site. Again, a consistent time-out procedure used throughout your organization is most effective.

TOOL

Surgical Safety Procedure Checklist

WHY DO I NEED TO KNOW THIS NOW?

High risk demands heightened attention. Standards related to high-risk procedures and the use of anesthesia span several chapters of the standards, and those related to the Universal Protocol are nested in the NPSG chapter.

WHERE DO I START?

- **Facilitate processes.** Review your organization's preanesthesia evaluation process to be sure it meets the standards and is consistently applied, depending on your deemed status. Work with clinical leaders to make it compliant, if necessary.
- **Conduct tracers.** To confirm that each step of the Universal Protocol is being implemented consistently for every relevant procedure, informally shadow several teams as they ready care recipients for procedures. In particular, check to be sure that the care recipient is involved in the process whenever possible.

KEY CONCEPT

SAFETY RISKS

Care recipient safety goes to the very core of the health care mission. Whether it's maintaining a safe environment of care, ensuring the safe delivery of care and services, or making sure that care recipients are well informed and can make informed decisions about their own care, identifying and eliminating—or minimizing—risks to safety should be a high organizational priority.

Identifying Care Recipients Correctly

A reliable system for correctly identifying care recipients is, of course, a critical safety tool. The risks that come with misidentification should be fairly obvious, including wrong-patient surgical procedures, medication errors, and newborns receiving breastmilk from the wrong postpartum patient, among others. A robust care recipient identification system uses at least two care recipient identifiers, excluding room number or physical location. Both identifiers should be checked whenever administering medication, performing procedures, delivering blood products, or taking samples. It is also required by NPSG.01.01.01, Element of Performance (EP) 2, to label specimens in the care recipient's presence to avoid confusion. Special care should be taken in the identification of newborns and other vulnerable care recipients.

Identifying Care Recipient Safety Risks

Because care recipient safety is so fundamental to achieving the mission of health care organizations, it is essential to have an organizationwide safety program serving care recipients. Establishing such a program is one way for leaders to promote a culture of safety across the organization. A designated safety manager or a cross-disciplinary team must create processes for identifying risks to care recipient safety, prioritizing risks, and designing changes in policies and procedures designed to limit or eliminate such risks. Risk assessment and after-action investigation of adverse and sentinel events should be done in a way that focuses on processes and policies, rather than individual culpability, which encourages frontline staff to look for and report perceived risks to care recipient safety.

just imagine...

Patient-Centered Communication

A nurse is explaining to a patient the possible side effects of a new medication. The patient nods occasionally but doesn't speak. When the nurse asks if she has any questions, the patient just nods again. The nurse suspects the patient doesn't understand the information, so the nurse gets a pen and paper to ask the patient if she understood. The patient shakes her head and writes something in Spanish. The nurse calls an interpreter to assist.

It's vital to be sure that the patient understands the information being shared. Identify the patient's communication needs, document in the health record, and communicate to staff. Various methods and technologies are useful for communicating with individuals who speak a language other than English or who are deaf or hard of hearing. These include in-person interpreters, qualified bilingual staff, or remote interpreting systems such as telephone or video interpreting, as well as the translation of written or braille materials.

WHY DO I NEED TO KNOW THIS NOW?

Keeping care recipients safe is essential to providing high-quality care. Without a safe environment of care and policies and procedures focused on care recipient safety, the organization cannot fulfill its mission. Further, Joint Commission standards require certain specific steps to ensure care recipient safety and that care is provided in a safe environment.

WHERE DO I START?

- Contact your organization's safety manager or team.
- Evaluate your organization's care recipient safety and care recipient identification programs.
- Ask frontline staff if they feel comfortable reporting perceived risks to care recipient safety. Ask if they feel their concerns are taken seriously and dealt with effectively.

KEY CONCEPT

RIGHTS AND RESPONSIBILITIES OF CARE RECIPIENTS

You care for the physical and mental health of care recipients. They know that because you show that. But do you show that you care about the rights of care recipients? And do you help make them aware of their responsibilities?

TOOL

Required Patient Rights and Responsibilities Checklist

Care Recipient Rights

Caring for care recipients must be done in a way that respects their rights. These rights include but aren't limited to the following:

- Privacy
- Informed consent
- Receiving health information in the manner most effective to the care recipient
- Participating in care decisions, including end-of-life decisions
- Having access to and information about how to make and pursue complaints about care and treatment

The Joint Commission requires organizations to have written policies regarding these rights—and care recipients need to be informed of them. Simply writing a list and a policy isn't enough. You must actively work to honor and promote those rights.

Interpreting and Translation

One of the rights of care recipients is the right to receive information in a manner they understand. This means your organization needs to provide language interpreting and translation services for care recipients with language barriers. You also need to accommodate care recipients with vision, speech, hearing, or cognitive variations.

Informed Consent and Advance Directives

For care recipients to be able to make informed decisions about their care, and participate in that care, they need to know about possible outcomes and risks of recommended care. They have the right to give or withhold informed consent or refuse care altogether. Advance directives related to end-of-life situations must be honored in accordance with organization policy.

Resolving Complaints

Care recipients also have the right to have their complaints reviewed by the organization. Your organization must have a process for addressing and resolving these complaints and a system for informing care recipients about that process.

For deemed status. You must provide the care recipient with details such as an organization contact person, time frame for review and response, and what steps were taken to investigate the complaint.

Care Recipient Responsibilities

Treating care recipients as active partners in their care requires communicating with them about their responsibilities. Assisted living communities, hospitals, home care organizations, and nursing care centers are required to have a written policy that is shared with care recipients that clearly outlines their responsibilities. These responsibilities may vary by setting and include but are not limited to the following:

- Providing accurate information to caregivers
- Asking questions or expressing that they don't understand
- Maintaining civil conduct and language
- Following instructions, policies, and rules to promote high-quality care and a safe environment for everyone
- Meeting financial responsibilities

Review the "Rights and Responsibilities of the Individual" (RI) chapter on E-dition or in your *Comprehensive Accreditation Manual* for more information related to care recipient responsibilities.

"I heard that...

organizations are bound to honor advance directives no matter what."

fact:

There may be cases in which a care recipient's advance directive goes against laws and regulations or is beyond your organization's capabilities. This information should be shared with care recipients.

Health Literacy

If care recipients don't understand the information they're given, their safety is at risk. Although an assessment of an individual's health literacy level is not a requirement, organizations must perform a learning needs assessment that includes physical and cognitive limitations and other barriers to communication. Organizations can develop easy-to-understand education materials and medication instruction to address the health literacy needs of its care recipient population(s).

WHY DO I NEED TO KNOW THIS NOW?

The care recipient–provider partnership is enhanced when individuals understand their responsibilities. Both sides need to understand what's expected in that partnership. Part of your work is building and supporting it.

WHERE DO I START?

- **Check documentation.** Evaluate your organization's policies that describe the rights and responsibilities of the care recipient—perhaps included in admission packets—including those for informed consent and advance directives and those for complaint review and resolution. How is information given in a manner the care recipient understands? Are your forms in order? Is documentation well organized and clear? How do your organization's policies address barriers to communication, such as the care recipient's cultural or religious beliefs, emotional barriers to understanding their desire and motivation to learn, physical or cognitive variations, or other barriers to communication?

CRITICAL CHALLENGES

Every year The Joint Commission publishes a list of standards that surveyors scored most often in the previous year. The list is broken down for each type of accreditation program, but many of these standards highlight issues that are challenging for all organizations. A review of the trends in these data shows two standards that might be challenging as you address the provision of care, treatment, and services in your organization.

CARE RECIPIENT PARTICIPATION

Often, noncompliance with standards for care plans has less to do with knowing what information should be in a care plan and more to do with making sure that information is in the care plan—including documentation of care recipient participation.

What's the problem? The data show that behavioral health care and human services organizations find it a challenge to comply with Standard CTS.03.01.03, which is about care plans:

- **In behavioral health care.** Compliance problems with this standard stem from not including documented contributions from the entire care team in the care plan—specifically, not including the care recipient's behavioral health care goals in the care recipient's own words.

WHY DO I NEED TO KNOW THIS NOW?

Care recipient involvement in health care requires education and participation. Both promote care recipient safety and minimize unintended harm. The Joint Commission needs to see documentation of that education and participation. If you support (and insist) on documented care recipient involvement starting now, other care recipient-centered compliance-related initiatives may be easier down the road.

WHERE DO I START?

- **Be a role model.** One method to get everyone involved in documenting care recipient education and participation is to form an interdisciplinary care recipient/family education group. The goals of this group might include the following:
  - Streamlining documentation to increase efficiency and minimize gaps and errors
  - Assessing documentation to make sure all aspects of care recipient/family education are being covered
  - Creating education documentation policies that apply to all disciplines
- **Conduct tracers.** Perform a tracer focused on care recipient education (it should cover multiple standards in multiple chapters).

SUICIDE ASSESSMENT

Because suicide attempts and acts of self-harm are commonly reported sentinel events, screening and assessment of care recipients for suicidality are required of behavioral health care programs and hospitals treating care recipients for psychiatric issues. It's not a bad idea to do an initial screening in other settings, given that many care recipients who attempt suicide have contact with the health care system within a year before the attempt, usually not for mental health reasons.

What's the problem? Under Standard NPSG.15.01.01, behavioral health care programs and hospitals treating care recipients for psychiatric issues must do an initial screening for suicidal ideation on all care recipients. Those care recipients who screen positive must be given an evidence-based suicide risk assessment. The Suicide Assessment Five-Step Evaluation and Triage (SAFE-T) and the Columbia Suicide Severity Rating Scale (C-SSRS) are available tools, but you should shop around for something that fits your organization and setting or create or adapt your own tool. The important thing is there must be evidence showing the tool's efficacy. The tool should cover the following indicators for elevated risk of self-harm:

- Suicidal ideation
- Plans
- Intent
- Suicidal or self-harm behaviors
- Risk factors
- Protective factors

TOOL

Suicide Prevention Assessment Checklist

Suicidality is a dynamic state, with ebbs and flows. Periodic reassessments can help practitioners evaluate the care recipient's risk of self-harm on an ongoing basis and make appropriate decisions regarding measures to keep high-risk care recipients safe. Such measures may include one-to-one monitoring, removing sharps and other dangerous objects from the care recipient's immediate vicinity, treating the care recipient in a room with ligature-resistant fixtures, or other measures deemed appropriate.

WHY DO I NEED TO KNOW THIS NOW?

Rising rates of opioid addiction, economic stress, and social isolation are driving higher rates of self-harm, and the availability of lethal means such as firearms is driving an increase in completed suicide attempts. As noted above, many people who die of suicide have contact with the health care system within a year beforehand. This gives health care professionals a unique opportunity to detect and assess care recipients' suicide risk and possibly intervene. Also, hospitals and other health care facilities can present a variety of environmental risks (ligature points, sharps, and so forth), and assessing care recipients for suicide risk is part of the overall care recipient safety effort.

WHERE DO I START?

- **Consult authorities.** There are many public health, academic, and professional organizations working on the problem of preventing suicide and care recipient suicide. State public health authorities, the US Centers for Disease Control and Prevention (CDC), and the Agency for Healthcare Research and Quality (AHRQ) are all good places to start. Many can provide you with basic tools and information to help you meet this challenge.
- **Screen, assess, and reassess.** So as not to overwhelm emergency department and other frontline staff, a short screener tool can be used to identify care recipients who should receive a full risk assessment. Assess those who screen positive and use the assessment to guide appropriate care decisions about supervision, treatment, and safety of the care recipient. Remember, suicidality is a dynamic condition. So you must regularly reassess care recipients' risk and alter supervision levels and other safety protocols accordingly.

Test Your Knowledge

1. Discharge planning is required only in hospital settings.
   - ☐ a. True
   - ☐ b. False

2. Which of the following is correct about care planning? (Select all that apply.)
   - ☐ a. It is individualized based on admission information.
   - ☐ b. It is required in all Joint Commission accredited programs, with the exception of the Laboratory and Point-of-Care Testing program.
   - ☐ c. It is required only for admissions longer than three days.
   - ☐ d. Documentation is optional.

3. Which of the following are considered by The Joint Commission to be high-risk or problem-prone clinical activities? (Select all that apply.)
   - ☐ a. Medication management
   - ☐ b. Operative/invasive procedures
   - ☐ c. Sedation/anesthesia
   - ☐ d. Restraint and seclusion

4. Care recipient responsibilities include meeting financial obligations with the organization.
   - ☐ a. True
   - ☐ b. False

5. Which of the follow statements about the National Patient Safety Goals (NPSG) is correct?
   - ☐ a. NPSGs are optional Joint Commission requirements.
   - ☐ b. NPSGs are the same for all Joint Commission accreditation programs.
   - ☐ c. NPSGs have not changed since their introduction in 2008.
   - ☐ d. The most frequently cited NPSGs in the Hospital program involve suicide risk.

Emergency Management

CHAPTER 10

THE BIG IDEA

Whether it's civil unrest, an infectious disease outbreak, a terrorist attack, or a geographic-specific concern, such as a hurricane, wildfire, earthquake, or tornado, all health care organizations need to be prepared for emergencies. Emergency management (EM) is, in fact, required for all Joint Commission accreditation programs, although the content of EM plans and specific concerns vary depending on your geographic area. The EM standards have been revised to better reflect the realities of the pandemic and other disasters with which health care organizations are dealing.

KEY CONCEPTS

- Framework for Preparedness
- Emergency Planning in Action

THE MANUAL

Following are the relevant Joint Commission E-dition® or *Comprehensive Accreditation Manual* chapters:

- "Environment of Care" (EC)
- "Emergency Management" (EM)
- "Equipment Management" (EQ) [home care only]
- "Life Safety" (LS) [not laboratory]

Note: *For home care settings, the LS standards and elements of performance (EPs) apply only to inpatient hospice.*

KEY CONCEPT

FRAMEWORK FOR PREPAREDNESS

To plan for and respond to emergencies effectively, you should understand the four phases of EM and how to address them. The four phases, along with Joint Commission standards, can help guide your planning and response efforts and help ensure that your plans are thorough and your response is robust and appropriate. In addition, remember to reach out to local agencies to ensure full compliance with all local, state, and federal requirements.

The Four Phases

One common thread—in health care and beyond—is the division of EM into four phases. Each phase includes a different set of activities with distinct purposes, as follows:

- **Mitigation.** Activities to reduce the severity and impact of a potential emergency
- **Preparedness.** Activities to build capacity and identify resources that may be used if an emergency occurs
- **Response.** Activities implemented to react to an emergency as it occurs
- **Recovery.** Activities to restore services after an emergency

Syncing with the community: Each phase should be integrated with your organization's community EM plan. All health care organizations in your community should collaborate on an overall emergency plan. First responders, the EM community (including regional organizations), and local and state health departments are all good starting points.

Hazard Vulnerability Analysis (HVA)

Emergency planning begins with a hazard vulnerability analysis (HVA). An HVA helps identify all potential internal and external hazards, emergencies, or events that your organization is likely to face or that will otherwise have an impact on your organization. The results of the HVA should help your organization's leaders assess probability of occurrence and probable impact. It'll also help you figure out your level of preparedness. The HVA should be developed with consideration of risks in the community and the community's capability to support the organization during an emergency.

Emergency Planning

Information from the HVA should then be used in the creation and annual evaluation of your emergency plan—known as either an emergency operations plan (EOP) or emergency management plan (EMP), depending on your organization's setting. An EOP and EMP must provide details about the critical capabilities that health care organizations need to address to protect care recipients, staff, and the facility during an emergency. These capabilities, also known as the six critical areas, are as follows:

1. Communications
2. Resources and assets
3. Security and safety
4. Staff responsibilities
5. Utilities
6. Patient [care recipient] clinical and support activities

An organization must have a comprehensive emergency management program that utilizes an all-hazards approach. The EM program must address leadership structure and program accountability, the HVA, mitigation and preparedness activities, the EOP/EMP and related policies and procedures (P&Ps), education and training, exercises and testing, a continuity of operations plan (COOP), disaster recovery, and program evaluation. An organization also should have someone designated as the emergency management leader for the organization.

Incident command system (ICS). Depending on the size of your organization, a vital part of the communications component in an EOP/EMP is an organized system of command and control. An ICS generally has five functional areas of control depending on the size of the planned or unplanned event (it can be expanded or contracted):

1. **Incident command.** Accountable for the incident response and provides identified priorities and strategies for the event
2. **Operations.** Establishes tactics and directs all operational resources
3. **Planning.** Supports the incident by tracking resources, collecting and analyzing data, and developing the Incident Action Plan
4. **Logistics.** Arranges resources and needed equipment to support the incident objectives (for example, personnel, supplies, equipment)
5. **Finance/administration.** Monitors all costs related to the incident and provides accounting and/or cost analysis

In addition, the ICS may include command staff who address public information, staff who address safety, and a government and private-sector liaison.

Emergency Exercises and Evaluation

Practice is part of emergency planning: All accredited organizations must conduct periodic emergency exercises. The exercises should meet the following criteria:

- Conducted on-site within your organization; and for some organizations, also as part of a communitywide exercise
- Tests the responsiveness of the organization to the effects of an emergency on its services, staffing, and facilities
- Demanding enough to reveal weaknesses, gaps, or opportunities for improvement in the organization's response efforts (that is, test to failure)
- Documented so results can then be reviewed, improvements applied, and any changes to the EOP/EMP can be made

TOOL

Emergency Response Staff Training Checklist

WHY DO I NEED TO KNOW THIS NOW?

When disaster strikes, there's no time to spare—health care organizations must be prepared to act. You need to help the staff prepare as an ongoing part of your job. And you must know whom to connect with and contact when an emergency emerges.

WHERE DO I START?

- **Work with leaders.** Treat emergency preparedness as an organizationwide responsibility. The organization's emergency management leader should establish an EM committee and involve key leaders which will lead to a successful emergency preparedness program. This committee not only establishes relationships and responsibilities within the organization, but it also establishes a centralized group to plan for emergency preparedness policy revisions, education, and training. Consider extending your committee meetings to include community EM officials, such as representatives from your local law enforcement and fire departments.
- **Work with staff.** Everyone in the organization has a role to play in an emergency. Talking with staff at all levels will help you assess the level of knowledge and understanding staff have of their roles in an emergency. You may also need to create training and education opportunities for staff to help them understand and perform their emergency roles.
- **Network with peers.** Work with colleagues at health care organizations in your community to share best practices, train together, and plan communitywide drills. This includes participating in local and/or regional EM meetings. Meetings of this nature provide guidance for understanding how to access regional or state cache and help define your organization's role and responsibilities during an event.
- **Participate in EM exercises.** Your organization's emergency management leader will develop EM exercises and drills as well as document and evaluate these exercises. Your role as accreditation professional includes supporting the EM leader as appropriate and necessary in these exercises in order to ensure compliance with Joint Commission standards.

KEY CONCEPT

EMERGENCY PLANNING IN ACTION

In an emergency your organization will need to communicate with a variety of individuals and organizations, from staff and care recipients, to state and local authorities, to community partners, to the media. Planning is essential to this complex task.

Establishing and Facilitating Communications

Given the complexity of the task of communicating during an emergency, it is very important to establish a communications policy that details who talks to whom and how. As part of your EM planning, your organization will establish an incident command center within your facility. All communications should issue from or be directed through the incident command center. The incident commander should designate a staff member to coordinate communications with staff within and outside the facility, local authorities and emergency managers, the media, the public, and others. This work includes specifying a means of communication (phones, text alerts, social media, intranet and Internet sites, ham radios, two-way radios) and ensuring that equipment is properly maintained, staff are

PICTURE THIS

Emergency Management Leader

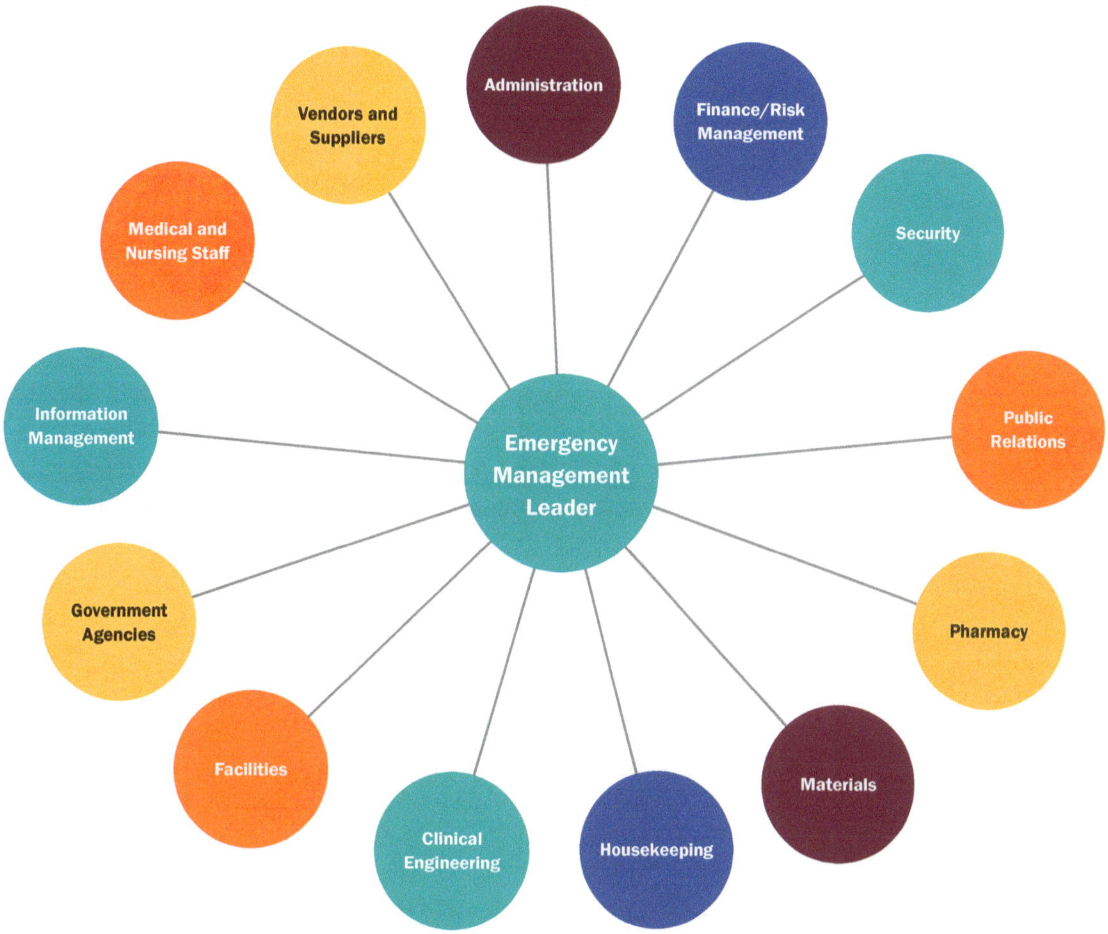

No matter the size of your organization, everyone has a role to play in the event of an emergency. Be sure to know who is involved in emergency management activities for your organization and participate as appropriate.

regularly trained to operate the equipment, and backup systems and plans are in place in case first-choice modes of communication are unavailable.

Plan B. No matter how well you prepare for emergencies, you cannot prepare for everything. Communication systems are susceptible to interruptions. Contacts may be unavailable. Equipment may be destroyed. Know ahead of time how you will respond to these challenges.

Managing Resources and Assets

In an emergency it is likely that the organization will experience supply chain and service disruptions that may cause shortages of medications, medical

THE 96-HOUR RULE

The Joint Commission requires all hospitals and nursing care centers to be able to assess capacity for operations without assistance for 96 hours. A comprehensive EOP describes ways the organization continues operations to deliver care to individuals during an emergency for up to 96 hours. One method to estimate your sustainability is to calculate the average daily census of care recipients by the routine consumption of resources and assets. In addition, ensure that reassessment of inventory at set intervals during an emergency is included in your emergency preparedness initiatives. This type of evaluation is typically for organizations that provide 24-hour inpatient care.

Note: *Health care organizations are not required to stockpile supplies to last 96 hours. However, during long-duration emergencies, an organization needs to monitor its capabilities and adjust its response procedures to support ongoing delivery of safe care.*

equipment and supplies, water, power, medical gas, or other resources. A detailed inventory of all critical organizational resources is an important tool for managing resources and assets in an emergency. The inventory should be maintained on an ongoing basis and it should include resources and supplies that are specifically dedicated for emergency use.

Your organization will need to work with vendors to plan for emergency delivery of needed supplies and equipment, including anticipating needs and logistical challenges. You should also cultivate relationships with alternative vendors, in case your usual vendor is overtaxed by demand or rendered unable to serve you in an emergency. For example, during one hurricane a supplier had all the trucks loaded, but the drivers had to evacuate, leaving hospital supplies in the delivery trucks at the warehouse. During the COVID-19 pandemic, similar to H1N1, N95 respirators and disinfecting wipes were on backorder around the world.

Staff Response

How will you alert on-site and off-site staff in an emergency? How will you inform them of critical information such as whether, when, and how to report to work? You will need detailed contact information for all staff. Keep this information current. Keep it in both electronic and hard-copy formats. Keep it in more than one place so that it will be accessible even if, for instance, your incident command center is inaccessible. It is also a good idea to have a way to alert staff quickly to an impending emergency and then direct them to a central clearinghouse for information, such as an intranet or Internet site dedicated to this purpose or a phone hotline; in addition, consider identifying a commercial radio and television station. You can then convey further information, such as staffing needs, road closures, and so on.

Managing your human resources. In a prolonged emergency, such as a natural disaster, it is easy for staff to get burned out by long hours, high operational tempo, stress, and emotional trauma. Plan how you are going to rotate staff, and make sure to give them access to counseling, mental health, and/or spiritual resources to help them remain healthy and effective. For example, your organization's plan may call for four-hour rotations in the command center for prolonged events such as flooding, hurricanes, or wildfires. Succession planning is key to ensuring that staff remain physically and mentally healthy.

Ensuring Safety and Security

Depending on the nature of the emergency, your organization may face special challenges in the areas of safety and security. Facilities may be damaged by earthquakes or high winds. Utility interruptions may cause blackouts. A cyberattack could shut down an emergency department. Large numbers of injured and/or panicked people may present themselves at a health care facility, such as a hospital or other health care location. The possibility of an active shooter situation must be considered.

To prepare for these and other possible challenges, you need a two-pronged approach. First, you will need to create a plan to communicate critical safety and security information within the facility. This includes evacuation procedures, lockdown protocols, ambulance diversions, and special changes to normal operations required by circumstances. You may use overhead codes or announcements, special signage, word of mouth spread via regular clinical or security rounds, or any other methods that seem necessary and effective. Limiting access—such as allowing entry only via specified doors—has worked well for some organizations. Make sure to consider how your organization will account for care recipient family members and whether you will badge them. Second, you will need to plan to communicate safety and security information to those outside your facility, such as police, fire officials, local emergency managers, and the public. Maintain relationships with local authorities and media organizations. When disaster strikes, you will want to convey accurate information quickly to relevant and concerned parties to facilitate emergency response and keep the public informed and calm.

Safeguarding Utilities

You can't deliver high-quality health care in the dark or without water—so your organization's physical building is the most important piece of equipment available. A key part of your mitigation activities should be identifying and prioritizing vulnerabilities in the systems that provide your facility with power; water; steam; and heating, ventilating, and air-conditioning (HVAC). Facilities staff can help with a review of existing systems to identify where they can be made safer from flooding, fire, sabotage, accidental damage, or other possible sources of interruption or damage.

Backup planning. Health care organizations—particularly hospitals—work with local utility companies to prioritize restoration of their services over other less critically important customers. Some plan with utility companies or outside vendors to deliver power generation trucks and/or tankers or potable and non-potable water to their facilities in the event these utilities are cut off for a substantial length of time. Many others use day or skid tanks to have on-site gasoline and diesel to keep the organization's fleet running (for example, lab couriers).

WHY DO I NEED TO KNOW THIS NOW?

Scarcity of resources is one of the biggest threats to an organization's ability to keep functioning in an emergency. Knowing what you have on hand and how and where to obtain more of what you need will help ease stress on the system.

WHERE DO I START?

- **Work with vendors.** Integrate your vendors into your EMP, and work with them to create plans for delivering critical supplies during an emergency; also include them in drills.
- **Know the location of the nearest CHEMPACK.** The US Administration for Strategic Preparedness and Response (ASPR) maintains strategically located stockpiles of nerve agent antidotes. In the event of a nerve agent release, you will need to know who to contact to access the CHEMPACK and statewide stockpiles.
- **Know what you are likely to need.** Use brainstorming, staff interviews, and exercises to learn what resources and assets are likely to be depleted in an emergency. Use this information to focus your emergency resource

TOOL

Emergency and Disaster Preparedness Evaluation Checklist

management planning efforts. For example, staff may use linens to stop horizontal water intrusion, therefore diminishing the supply of clean linens.

- **Stockpile critical supplies.** Be sure that you have strategic stockpiles of critical supplies on-site, in case deliveries are delayed.

CRITICAL CHALLENGES

Every year The Joint Commission publishes a list of standards that surveyors scored most often in the previous year. The list is broken down for each type of accreditation program, but many of these standards highlight issues that are challenging for all organizations. A review of the trends in these data shows a standard that might be challenging as you address emergency management in your organization.

TOOL

Emergency Planning Evaluation Checklist

POLICY/PROCEDURE FOR REQUESTING AN 1135 WAIVER

For deemed status: According to Standard EM.12.01.01, Element of Performance (EP) 9, hospitals and critical access hospitals using Joint Commission accreditation for deemed status with the US Centers for Medicare & Medicaid Services (CMS) must have policies and procedures in place for the requesting of 1135 waivers. (**You do not have to have a waiver for survey.**) These waivers relax certain requirements of CMS programs for a defined period of time after a disaster declaration. This may include permitting program participants to receive care at alternative care sites defined by emergency managers.

What's the problem? Depending on the population your organization serves, as well as your organization's setting and community, you will need to assess what kinds of 1135 waivers you might need. It is a good idea to have standard 1135 waiver request paperwork on hand in the incident command center and to fill out appropriate request forms to the degree possible in advance. You will also need to know who has the authority to request 1135 waivers and who is responsible for filling out and transmitting requests.

WHY DO I NEED TO KNOW THIS NOW?

Organizations must have policies and procedures in place to request an 1135 waiver. Having this documentation is a Joint Commission requirement, but more importantly, confirming that this documentation is in place will facilitate the request process when an emergency is declared and an 1135 waiver needs to be submitted to CMS.

WHERE DO I START?

- **Be informed.** As the accreditation professional for your organization, you need to ensure compliance with all Joint Commission requirements. Review the policy and procedure to ensure that it is current in accordance with your organization's policy review schedule.

- **Understand the process.** Know what is required when submitting an 1135 waiver and how to prepare and submit a waiver. Know who is responsible for requesting these waivers or who is authorized to approve and sign off on a waiver request.

Test Your Knowledge

1. Match the phrase with the definition.

Activities to restore services	Mitigation
Activities to build capacity	Response
Activities to lessen impact	Recovery
Activities implemented to react	Preparedness

2. The proactive risk assessment emergency management tool for determining severity, criticality, and frequency of potential emergencies or disasters is called ___.
   - ☐ a. failure mode and effects analysis
   - ☐ b. root cause analysis
   - ☐ c. hazard vulnerability analysis
   - ☐ d. sentinel event

3. Which of the following are correct statements about 1135 waivers?
   - ☐ a. After the individual or team responsible for emergency management approves your 1135 waiver, you are ready to go.
   - ☐ b. When an 1135 waiver is approved, it is effective for three months.
   - ☐ c. A Centers for Medicare & Medicaid Services regional office must approve an 1135 waiver.
   - ☐ d. The Joint Commission must approve an 1135 waiver.

4. According to Joint Commission requirements, how long should your emergency operations plan be able to cover your operations?
   - ☐ a. 48 hours
   - ☐ b. 72 hours
   - ☐ c. 96 hours
   - ☐ d. 144 hours

Environment of Care

CHAPTER 11

THE BIG IDEA

The physical environment of a health care organization (its buildings, utilities, medical equipment, and more) is known as the environment of care (EC). A safe physical environment is vital to the safe care and treatment of care recipients and the safety and security of everyone in the facility: staff, care recipients, contract workers, and visitors. It's also the right—and responsibility—of everyone in the facility.

KEY CONCEPTS

- Management Plans
- Risk Assessments
- Hazardous Materials and Waste
- Safety and Security
- Medical Equipment and Utilities

THE MANUAL

Following are the relevant Joint Commission E-dition® or *Comprehensive Accreditation Manual* chapters:

- "Emergency Management" (EM)
- "Environment of Care" (EC)
- "Equipment Management" (EQ) [home care only]
- "Life Safety" (LS) [not laboratory]

Top Challenging Environment of Care Standards

These standards and EPs are those EC requirements that have recently been most frequently cited by surveyors as being non-compliant.

Standard	Element of Performance (EP)	Applicable Accreditation Program(s)
EC.02.02.01: The organization manages risks related to hazardous materials and waste.	**EP 5:** The organization minimizes risks associated with selecting, handling, storing, transporting, using, and disposing of hazardous chemicals.	Ambulatory Care, Critical Access Hospital, Hospital, Nursing Care Center
EC.02.04.03: The laboratory inspects, tests, and maintains laboratory equipment.	**EP 7:** The laboratory performs preventive maintenance, periodic inspection, and performance testing of each instrument or piece of equipment. These activities are documented.	Laboratory
EC.02.05.01: The organization manages risks associated with its utility systems.	**EP 7:** In areas assigned to control airborne contaminants (such as biological agents, gases, fumes, dust), the ventilation systems provide appropriate pressure relationships, air-exchange rates, filtration efficiencies, relative humidity, and temperature.	Ambulatory Care
EC.02.05.01: The organization manages risks associated with its utility systems.	**EP 15:** In critical care areas designed to control airborne contaminants (such as biological agents, gases, fumes, dust), the ventilation system provides appropriate pressure relationships, air-exchange rates, filtration efficiencies, temperature, and humidity. For new and existing health care facilities, or altered, renovated, or modernized portions of existing systems or individual components (constructed or plans approved on or after July 5, 2016), heating, cooling, and ventilation are in accordance with NFPA 99-2012, which includes 2008 ASHRAE 170, or state design requirements if more stringent.	Critical Access Hospital, Hospital
EC.02.06.01: The organization establishes and maintains a safe, functional environment.	**EP 1:** Interior spaces meet the needs of the patient population and are safe and suitable to the care, treatment, and services provided.	Hospital, Nursing Care Center, Office-Based Surgery

KEY CONCEPT

MANAGEMENT PLANS

To make effective and sustained improvements in the clinical arena, you need to implement plans based on reducing identified risks. It's a very similar process in the nonclinical arena.

Required Management Plans

The Joint Commission requires management plans for six functional areas covered by the EC chapter:

1. Safety
2. Security
3. Hazardous materials and waste
4. Fire safety
5. Medical equipment
6. Utilities

Focus and development. Management plans focus on risk management—identifying risks and then minimizing or eliminating them. The plans may be developed by the person(s) identified to manage and reduce risks or by an EC committee. Ideally, these plans should be developed by an interdisciplinary team.

Scope and depth. EC management plans should cover all organization sites, summarize how relevant standards and elements of performance (EPs) are met, and identify those responsible for completing specific tasks within required time frames. Although comprehensive in scope, they are high-level plans, such as executive summaries, not operational plans. Surveyors assess the plans on scope, objectives, performance, and effectiveness.

WHY DO I NEED TO KNOW THIS NOW?

Management plans are based on the EC standards. And you'll be more on top of what's happening during the environmental tours. Note that environmental tours are not a Joint Commission requirement for most organizations. However, they can help organizations identify hazardous conditions, observe safety practices and behaviors, eliminate potential hazards, and monitor staff knowledge. Also, during your Joint Commission survey, the surveyor will conduct interviews to review staff understanding and implementation of the management plans.

WHERE DO I START?

- **Collaborate with experts.** Meet with relevant staff or committees to review all EC management plans. Get to know your facility manager(s) and other EC and life safety experts at your organization. You will work closely with these professionals to maintain your accreditation compliance.

PRIORITY

Sustainable Healthcare

The increasing severity of climate-based events affects health care organizations' operations as they face disruptions in care and challenges in patient safety. Extreme climate-based events also exacerbate chronic cardiac, respiratory, and other conditions, which are particularly acute for those who are at a socioeconomic, racial, ethnic, or geographic disadvantage, making climate change a health equity problem as well.

Many health systems are on their way to becoming more resilient to the effects of climate change. Cost savings may be realized by utilizing energy-efficient technologies, implementing waste management strategies, and taking advantage of the climate provisions in recently enacted federal law, which allow for new or expanded tax credits for energy-efficient facilities and incentives for equipment that can be used for renewable energy.

Many health care organizations are looking for a framework to help leaders and governance set priorities, as well as to develop skills to reduce waste and their carbon footprint. To answer this call, The Joint Commission has developed two resources specifically

(continued)

TOOLS

Sustainable Healthcare Certification Checklist

EC Management Plan Evaluation Checklist

Environmental Tour Checklist

(continued)

aimed at reducing emissions: the Sustainable Healthcare Certification Resource Center and the Sustainable Healthcare Certification program. Find easy-to-use tools, literature, videos and links in the Sustainable Healthcare Certification Resource Center section on The Joint Commission's website.

Sustainable Healthcare Certification is available to both accredited and nonaccredited US hospitals and critical access hospitals. The certification provides a framework to help organizations expand or continue their decarbonization efforts and receive public recognition for their commitment to sustainability.

KEY CONCEPT

RISK ASSESSMENTS

An EC management plan is only as strong as the risk assessment it was developed to meet. Joint Commission EC standards require organizations to identify safety and security risks in the EC that may affect care recipients, staff, or visitors. For the risk assessments that can be used, *see* the "Environment of Care" (EC) chapter on E-dition or in your book or e-book version of the *Comprehensive Accreditation Manual*. In addition, preconstruction and infection control risk assessments are required prior to construction projects (see Chapter 13 for additional information related to infection prevention and control). Risks may be identified from internal sources such as ongoing monitoring of the environment, results of root cause analyses, results of proactive risk assessments of high-risk processes, and from credible external sources such as *Sentinel Event Alerts*.

Standardized approach. If you use a standardized risk assessment approach for issues discovered on environmental tours, the process will go more smoothly because everyone knows "what's next." This is one possible standardized approach:

Step 1. Identify the issue.
Step 2. Develop arguments that support the proposed process or issue.
Step 3. Develop arguments against the proposed process or issue.
Step 4. Evaluate the arguments.
Step 5. Reach a conclusion.
Step 6. Document the process.
Step 7. Monitor and reassess the conclusion.

Environmental Tours

Risks are typically identified during environmental tours, sometimes called surveillance checks, which are based on the environmental management plans. Although not required by The Joint Commission, these tours can be used for assessing everyday risks as well as for monitoring compliance in general. Frequency should be determined by the organization.

WHY DO I NEED TO KNOW THIS NOW?

Risk assessments are tools that help identify areas for improvement or areas to watch for potential issues in the future. Keeping the physical environment safe is critical for your organization to provide high-quality care, treatment, and services.

WHERE DO I START?

- **Participate in environmental tours.** Go along on tours to determine the presence of unsafe conditions and ascertain whether your organization's current processes for managing environmental safety risks are practiced correctly and are effective. Follow up on plans developed to address each compliance violation or risk discovered (see Chapters 5 and 6).

PICTURE THIS

Everyday EC Risks

Buildings

workplace violence, internal fires, natural disasters, property/grounds damage

Equipment

defects, recalls, operating errors, ground fault, battery failures

Employees

infectious disease, hazardous materials, slips/trips/falls, burns, back injuries, needlesticks, electric shock, noise

Care Recipients and the Public

elevator malfunction, family violence, roadways/walkways/byways

- **Use tracers.** Consider conducting tracers on a regular or ad hoc basis. Topics may be related to issues identified during environmental tours that need further risk assessment or analysis or may encompass various areas of compliance (for example, EC, infection control) for evaluation. Make sure to use an interdisciplinary team and work with relevant EC staff to craft an action plan for any issues you discover.

TOOL

Environment of Care Rounds Assessment Checklist

PICTURE THIS

Environment of Care–Related *Sentinel Event Alerts*

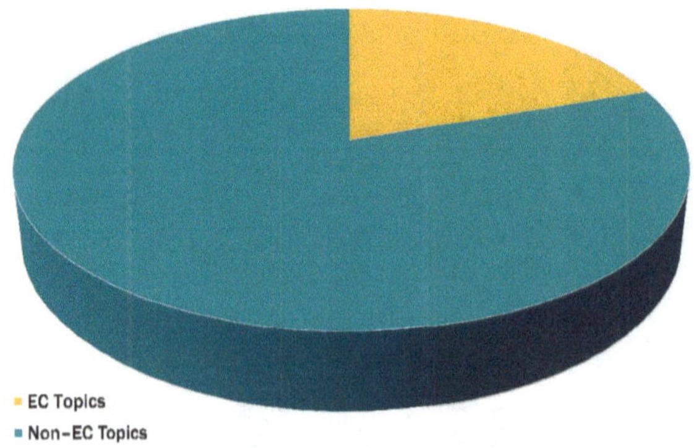

#9 **Infant abductions**
#15 **Infusion pumps**
#22 **Needlestick and sharps injuries**
#29 **Surgical fires**
#37 **Emergency electrical power system failures**
#45 **Violence in the health care setting**
#46 **Suicide in medical/surgical units and the emergency department**
#47 **Radiation risks of diagnostic imaging**
#50 **Medical device alarm safety**
#54 **Safe use of health information technology**
#56 **Detecting and treating suicidal ideation**
#59 **Physical and verbal violence toward health care workers**
#68 **Updating surgical fire prevention for the 21st century**

Of The Joint Commission's 68 *Sentinel Event Alerts*, 13 are on topics related to the environment of care (EC). Sentinel events are not only events that occur during the care and treatment of individuals. Physical and verbal violence, abductions, and power failures are all potential sentinel events that can affect your organization.

KEY CONCEPT

HAZARDOUS MATERIALS AND WASTE

"From cradle to grave." That's the commitment for managing hazardous materials and waste, or hazmat. In other words, to be compliant, you must manage hazardous materials and waste from the time they enter the facility to the time at which they're finally disposed of. That responsibility encompasses the following procedures:

- Selecting
- Handling
- Labeling
- Storing
- Transporting
- Using
- Generating
- Monitoring
- Disposing
- Documenting
- Staff training

Contracted services. If you use contracted services for hazardous materials and waste, your organization is still ultimately responsible: You have to make sure your vendor meets Joint Commission standards and other laws and regulations. That includes proper licenses, permits, and manifests.

Hazmat Inventory

With potentially deadly materials, you'd better know exactly what you're dealing with. For that reason, your organization must have an up-to-date written inventory of hazardous materials and waste. Note: The inventory only needs to include hazmat addressed by law and regulation, including those of the US Occupational Safety and Health Administration (OSHA), the US Environmental Protection Agency (EPA), the US Department of Transportation (DOT), and state and local laws and regulations.

Spills and Exposures

Hazmat procedures should minimize the risks of exposure to a hazardous materials spill or release (for example, a formaldehyde spill or a nitrous oxide gas leak). To minimize the risk of exposure, staff should be trained on the proper use of personal protective equipment (PPE), engineering controls (such as ventilation, alarms, and so forth), spill kits, and escalation procedures (that is, fire department, outside spill response team, emergency operations plan [EOP]/ emergency management plan [EMP], and so forth). Develop the procedures in advance of any hazmat emergency.

Responding to incidents. The standards require written procedures for responding to a hazmat incident. These should include procedures for alerting trained internal or external responders, containment and disposal of the material, and reporting the incident.

Safety Data Sheets

Staff must know about hazardous materials and waste within your facilities. And organizations must have a safety data sheet (SDS) for each hazardous material in the inventory. OSHA requires that these SDSs be accessible to all staff.

Chemical Inventory

Per OSHA, which EPA references for chemical inventory requirements, the minimal chemical inventory should contain the following:

- **Chemical name.** This information includes the complete name that is on the label, as well as the common name, synonyms, product/mixture name (if applicable), and percentage of ingredients in product/mixture (if applicable).
- **Manufacturer name.** Company name that produced the chemical and the name of the vendor who sold it
- **SDS on file.** An SDS is required for each item on this list.
- **CAS/catalog number.** The number assigned by the Chemical Abstracts Service (CAS) or the product number in a materials catalog
- **Quantity and estimated weight/volume.** Maximum number of each chemical as well as total approximate weight/volume of the chemicals on hand in your organization

- **Location.** Identify where the chemical is in your facility.
- **Hazards and PPE.** This list should include any health, safety, or fire risks as noted on the SDS, as well as any PPE required for handling the chemical.
- **Training.** Describe the training required to handle the chemical, as applicable.

DOT does not require a chemical inventory because its focus is on the shipment of the hazardous materials (that is, manifests). But because The Joint Commission requires that your hazardous waste be included on your inventory, the use of the DOT United Nations (UN) number would be an acceptable identifier for this hazardous waste if no CAS number is available.

"I heard that...

when our organization receives a delivery of radioactive material, we're required to have a security escort for the delivery person."

fact:

A security escort is not required by The Joint Commission or the Nuclear Regulatory Commission. However, some organizations choose to take this measure. If your organization's policy says that an escort is necessary, then a surveyor will check to see if you're complying with your own policy. Also, the person delivering radioactive materials must be a radiation worker, with specific training and credentials.

WHY DO I NEED TO KNOW THIS NOW?

An increasingly wide range of health care practices involve hazardous materials, with clinical and nonclinical staff at risk of exposure. Also, much of the hazmat documentation required by The Joint Commission is also required by other laws and regulations, so complying with The Joint Commission will help you comply with those as well.

WHERE DO I START?

- **Review documents.** Review your hazmat inventory (as a new accreditation professional and then annually after that) with relevant staff—facility manager, safety officer, materials management staff. Make sure the inventory format is consistent across departments, particularly in descriptions of each product/chemical and the definitions of the types of hazardous materials and waste (chemicals, chemotherapeutic agents, radioactive agents).

KEY CONCEPT

SAFETY AND SECURITY

Safety and security are often mentioned together when discussing the EC standards. But each must have its own management plan because each addresses a different type of risk.

Safety

These requirements address risks usually related to accidental incidents that occur in everyday tasks, in the physical structure, or due to uncontrollable factors such as weather. For that reason, the safety management plan should also cover worker safety—reducing the risk of worker injuries and occupational illness.

A healthy environment. General goals of a healthy environment, such as prohibiting smoking, ensuring adequate lighting, and controlling noise levels, also fall under the safety plan purview.

Security

These requirements address risks related to incidents that are often intentional and result in harm or loss to people and property (workplace violence, including shootings; care recipient suicides; bomb threats; care recipient wanderings or elopements; infant or pediatric abductions; drug thefts). The security management plan should include system procedures for all those security risks and others your organization has identified.

TOOL

Security Risk Analysis Form

Controlling access. The standards for most organizations require identifying people entering the facility. All organizations must control access to security-sensitive areas (as identified based on your risk assessment), such as the newborn nursery, the pharmacy, health records, or the emergency department.

Job Hazards Analysis

To help ensure the safety of health care workers in your organization, you should perform a job hazards analysis for each job or job category in your organization. Although not required by Joint Commission standards, this kind of analysis is required by OSHA. The Joint Commission does require each hospital and critical access hospital to conduct an annual worksite analysis of its workplace violence prevention program.

Work with staff through interviews and observation to break their duties down into individual steps. Then help them identify the steps or activities with the highest risk. With this information you can help devise strategies for minimizing or eliminating those risks.

Document it. In addition to interviewing the staff member working a particular job, it may be useful to record video of the worker performing their duties. Also, interviewing others who have done that job previously may produce valuable insights.

WHY DO I NEED TO KNOW THIS NOW?

Safety and security risks need everyday vigilance and awareness to remain in compliance and to protect everyone in the organization. You need to be aware of these risks every day.

WHERE DO I START?

- **Attend and observe.** Get to know your organization's safety officer (if you have one) and ask to job shadow for a few hours a month.
- **Provide education.** Make sure everyone is aware of safety and security risks and how to respond to incidents according to your organization's policies and procedures. Perhaps conduct a training session on how to complete your organization's incident reports, using examples of events. Be sure to address any gaps in staff training on dealing with workplace violence. The Joint Commission hosts a workplace violence prevention portal on its website to support organizations in preventing, preparing for, and mitigating the impact of, workplace violence.
- **Assess risks.** Perform a risk assessment for environmental factors in suicide risk. This can be critical within non-behavioral health care units and emergency rooms, which have had increasing incidents in this area.

Ready-to-use tools are available from OSHA, The Joint Commission's website, and organizations such as the Emergency Nurses Association.

KEY CONCEPT

MEDICAL EQUIPMENT AND UTILITIES

It's hard to imagine the modern health care environment without medical equipment like smart pumps. And how healthy could it be without utilities providing clean air? But just having medical equipment and utilities isn't enough: Joint Commission standards require that you manage risks for these integral EC and EQ (for home care only) components and ensure that they're in good working order.

What exactly are medical equipment and utilities, in the view of The Joint Commission?

- **Medical equipment.** This includes equipment used in monitoring, treatment, diagnosis, or direct care of care recipients (it excludes personal items, such as mobile phones).
- **Utilities.** This includes but is not limited to electrical distribution; emergency power; vertical and horizontal transport; HVAC (heating, ventilating, and air-conditioning); plumbing, boiler and steam systems, piped medical gas; vacuum systems; and communication systems.

Collaborative Management

Management of medical equipment requires a collaboration between clinical engineering staff and end users:

- Providers need to understand the operation.
- Engineering staff need to understand the maintenance.
- Both should understand application of equipment in the organization.

Utilities management requires the same kind of collaboration but has additional considerations, such as infection control issues.

Testing and Maintenance

Joint Commission standards require organizations to follow defined activities and frequencies for inspecting, testing, and maintaining medical equipment and utilities systems. To be prepared for maintenance discussions with EC staff, keep these concepts in mind:

- **Maintenance activities.** These preventive activities are based on the likely failure modes of the equipment or utilities (as identified through a maintenance strategy) and normal wear and tear.
- **Maintenance strategies.** These include interval-based (per the calendar), planned predictive (per status/performance testing), metered (per run time or usage), reliability-centered (per industry track records), and corrective (repaired or replaced upon failure) maintenance. The required intervals for interval-based maintenance are defined by The Joint Commission as follows:

- Daily = every day, once per day
- Weekly = every week, once per week
- Monthly = every month, once per month
- Quarterly = every 3 months, +/− 10 days
- Semiannual = 6 months from the last scheduled event, +/− 20 days
- Annual = 12 months from the last scheduled event, +/− 30 days
- Three years = 36 months from the last scheduled event, +/− 45 days

For deemed status. The US Centers for Medicare & Medicaid Services (CMS) requires that all equipment maintenance for health care organizations follow manufacturer's guidelines, in contrast to more flexibility provided by The Joint Commission in creating maintenance plans. CMS may in some circumstances allow you to develop and follow a customized alternative equipment maintenance (AEM) program, provided it does not compromise equipment safety. Be aware of current Survey and Certification memos from CMS and how they may apply to your organization.

WHY DO I NEED TO KNOW THIS NOW?

In your accreditation management role, you serve as liaison between EC staff and clinical care staff. You can start now, during the routine use of medical equipment and utilities, to help both groups understand the benefits of effective interactive management of EC.

WHERE DO I START?

- **Review documents.** Review the medical equipment and utility inventory and the process for determining the activities and frequencies related to inspections, testing, and maintenance of the equipment. Ensure that labels, maps, and other shared information are clear to non-EC staff.
- **Provide education.** If materials don't already exist, pull together information to educate staff on the proper use of the equipment, reporting malfunctioning equipment, and intervention/emergency procedures. Another important topic that pulls together EC and clinical operations is clinical alarms, the topic of a National Patient Safety Goal (NPSG).
- **Collaborate with experts.** Review human resources (HR) training records and work with HR and EC staff to make sure that end users know how to use equipment and how to respond to failure of equipment and utilities.
- **Check documentation.** Check that required documentation exists for the following: (1) procedures for inspecting, testing, and maintaining the equipment; (2) criteria for the AEM program; (3) person developing AEM program is qualified; (4) evidence of following those procedures and corrective actions; and (5) emergency procedures and response.

CRITICAL CHALLENGES

Every year The Joint Commission publishes a list of standards that surveyors scored most often in the previous year. The list is broken down for each type of accreditation program, but many of these standards highlight issues that are challenging for all organizations. A review of the trends in these data shows two standards that might be challenging as you address environment of care issues in your organization.

TESTING REQUIREMENTS

The Joint Commission doesn't mandate any specific fire alarm system, but Standard EC.02.03.05 lays out a rigorous testing schedule for facilities' fire alarm systems.

What's the problem? Fire alarm and suppression systems can be very complex and involve lots of different components. Some organizations struggle to devise and stick to a maintenance and testing schedule that takes in the entire system and all its component parts.

WHY DO I NEED TO KNOW THIS NOW?

Maintaining fire alarm and suppression systems is critical to keeping your organization safe in the event of a fire. Work with facilities staff to develop a schedule that tests the entire fire alarm and suppression system, as well as a maintenance schedule, to comply with Standard EC.02.03.05.

WHERE DO I START?

- Identify a schedule. Identify what the testing and maintenance schedule is for your organization's fire alarm and suppression systems. If this is an issue your organization has been cited for, work with facilities staff to find solutions that will bring your organization into compliance.
- Work with staff. Ensure that inspection and testing intervals are kept current by working with maintenance staff and servicing vendors.

SELF-HARM AND LIGATURE ISSUES

Part of providing an environment that is safe and suitable to the care, treatment, and services provided to the population of care recipients is identifying and eliminating or mitigating ligature risks or other potential risks leading to self-harm in the environment of care. This is particularly important in behavioral health care settings and general hospitals where care recipients may be treated for psychiatric issues, as these care recipients may be at elevated risk for suicide.

One quarter of Joint Commission–accredited behavioral health care and human services organizations are noncompliant with Standard NPSG.15.01.01, which includes a requirement to conduct a risk assessment of the physical environment (including storage space, waiting and reception areas, restrooms, lighting, and so on) to identify features that could be used to attempt suicide, and taking action to minimize the risk(s).

What's the problem? Some Requirements for Improvement (RFIs) come from overlooked environmental suicide risks, such as exposed plumbing in psychiatric units. Emphasis on identifying ligature risks is an important part of environmental rounds; however, ensure that staff tasked to identify these risks have the necessary experience to complete this task.

WHY DO I NEED TO KNOW THIS NOW?

Being able to provide safe, high-quality care and treatment requires a safe physical environment for care recipients. Ensuring that ligature risks are eliminated or mitigated is a critical component to maintaining a safe environment.

WHERE DO I START?

- **Participate in environmental tours.** Participating in environmental tours is an excellent way to see all aspects of your organization and to focus on identifying ligature risks.
- **Talk with staff.** Some areas of your organization may be more adept at addressing ligature risks than others. Talk with staff who address this concern often and with staff who do not. Share lessons learned and discuss ideas to ensure that ligature risks are properly eliminated or mitigated in all areas of your organization.

TOOL

Environmental Risks for Suicide Assessment Checklist

Test Your Knowledge

1. The Joint Commission requires organizations to include the six functional areas covered by the EC chapter into management plans.
   - ☐ a. True
   - ☐ b. False
2. The Joint Commission requires all health care organizations to do environmental tours.
   - ☐ a. True
   - ☐ b. False
3. Which of the following statements are true? (Select all that apply.)
   - ☐ a. If you have hazardous materials in your organization, you need to address exposures and spills in your plan.
   - ☐ b. If you contract with a vendor for hazardous waste removal, no further requirements are needed by your organization.
   - ☐ c. Safety data sheets are needed for all hazardous materials in your organization.
4. Based on Joint Commission requirements, workplace injuries are ___ issues.
   - ☐ a. compliance
   - ☐ b. safety
   - ☐ c. security
   - ☐ d. wellness
5. Which of the following statements are true? (Select all that apply.)
   - ☐ a. Equipment maintained by a vendor is not in the scope of your biomedical equipment plan.
   - ☐ b. The utilities plan must stipulate which individual(s) can turn off medical gas wall valves.
   - ☐ c. Your management plans must be reviewed every year.
   - ☐ d. Your organization's accreditation lead owns the environment of care management plan.

Fire Safety and Life Safety

CHAPTER 12

THE BIG IDEA

Fire protection is about preventing injury to life and/or property damage as a result of smoke, fire, and combustion. It's based on the "unit concept," which is basically that fire and products of combustion should be contained in the smallest compartment possible to prevent the spread of smoke and fire throughout the facility. Fire safety and life safety both relate to fire protection, but they differ for the purposes of Joint Commission requirements:

- **Fire safety.** Fire protection that is dependent on human intervention. Conducting fire drills, using fire safety equipment (fire extinguishers and pull stations), and maintaining means of egress and fire exits are part of fire safety. Requirements covering fire safety are in the "Environment of Care" (EC) chapter.
- **Life safety.** Fire protection dependent on building features. This includes alarm and sprinkler systems, construction, building design (including exits), and hardware issues. These requirements are in the "Life Safety" (LS) chapter.

KEY CONCEPTS

- Fire Safety and Life Safety Responsibilities
- Assessing Risks
- Interim Life Safety Measures

THE MANUAL

Following are the relevant Joint Commission E-dition® or *Comprehensive Accreditation Manual* chapters:

- "Environment of Care" (EC)
- "Life Safety" (LS) [not laboratory]

KEY CONCEPT

FIRE SAFETY AND LIFE SAFETY RESPONSIBILITIES

Fire safety and life safety requirements both relate to fire protection, and maintaining compliance is critical for your organization. Fire safety and life safety are interrelated, but they do differ from each other.

Fire Safety Responsibilities

As the accreditation professional for your organization, you need to be aware of the Joint Commission fire safety–related requirements to gauge whether your organization is compliant. Make sure that staff assigned to plan and conduct fire drills and maintain fire safety equipment are familiar with the requirements for the following two tasks that are critical to maintaining fire safety:

TOOL

Fire Drill Matrix

Fire drills. Standard EC.02.03.03 requires all health care organizations to conduct fire drills. Involve all staff, including licensed practitioners, volunteers, students, and contract staff (whether temporary or full-time), in fire drills. Vary the times and days of drills (a minimum of one hour apart) to ensure that all staff on all shifts practice their roles. Also, don't forget to include the operating room, the kitchen (most fires occur with cooking equipment), and the MRI suite in fire drills.

Fire safety equipment. As with medical equipment, EC fire safety standards require organizations to perform maintenance, inspection, and testing of fire safety equipment—and to document it. In addition, staff need to know their roles and responsibilities, including the proper use of fire safety equipment.

Life Safety Responsibilities

If you know your organization has life safety deficiencies (which can be identified by conducting your own optional environmental tours or mock tracers or in your recent accreditation findings), the logical next step is to address them and document how they're being managed. But first you need to understand the deficiencies in terms of the LS standards—and how those relate to requirements defined by the National Fire Protection Association (NFPA). Important concepts include the following:

LS Chapter and the *Life Safety Code*®.* The standards in the LS chapter are based on the 2012 edition of the *Life Safety Code*, issued by the NFPA. Each element of performance (EP) of the LS standards includes a reference to a section of the *Life Safety Code*. The US Centers for Medicare & Medicaid Services (CMS) Conditions of Participation (CoPs) are now aligned with provisions of the 2012 *Life Safety Code* too.

---

* *Life Safety Code*® is a registered trademark of the National Fire Protection Association, Quincy, MA.

Occupancy type. The LS requirements are based on occupancy, as defined by the NFPA (see the chart that follows). Occupant protection strategy differs by occupancy type; for example, health care occupancies are expected to "defend in place," while business occupancies must evacuate immediately.

Statement of Conditions™ (SOC). The SOC is an electronic tool, available on your *Joint Commission Connect®* extranet site, to help you assess your building's compliance with LS standards. In accordance with the requirements of Standard LS.01.01.01, an organization must assign an individual to manage the SOC when addressing survey-related deficiencies. The SOC has four parts, or tabs:

1. **Basic Building Information (BBI).** This is a demographic review of building occupancies and related information from your organization's electronic application for accreditation (E-App).
2. **Plans for Improvement (PFIs).** This optional tab allows the organization to capture plans for managing and correcting self-identified EC and LS deficiencies and to maintain continuous compliance.
3. **Survey-Related Plans for Improvement (SPFIs).** An SPFI is required only when an organization submits a Time-Limited Waiver or Equivalency Request. The SPFI must identify the corrective actions the organization has taken to show Evidence of Standards Compliance (ESC). If the actions

Life Safety Occupancy Types (as defined in Chapter 3 of the 2012 *Life Safety Code* by the National Fire Protection Association)	
Ambulatory care	Provides services or treatment on an outpatient basis to four or more* patients at the same time, in which the treatment or anesthesia renders patients incapable of self-preservation without assistance in an emergency; or provides urgent care for patients who, due to the nature of their injury or illness, are incapable of the same.
Business	Provides outpatient care, treatment, day treatment, or other services that do not meet the criteria in the ambulatory health care occupancy definition (for example, three or fewer* individuals at the same time who are either rendered incapable of self-preservation in an emergency or are undergoing general anesthesia).
Health care	For purposes such as medical or other treatment or care of persons suffering from physical or mental illness, disease, or infirmity; and for the care of infants, convalescents, or infirm aged persons. Health care occupancies provide sleeping facilities for four or more occupants and are occupied by persons who are mostly incapable of self-preservation because of age, physical or mental disability, or security measures not under the occupant's control. Health care occupancies include hospitals, critical care access hospitals, skilled nursing homes, and limited care facilities.
Residential	Provides sleeping accommodations for normal residential purposes and includes all buildings designed to provide sleeping accommodations.

* For CMS deemed ambulatory surgical centers, the definition applies when one or more care recipients is provided services.

needed to correct the deficiencies will exceed the 60-day time frame, the organization must request a time-limited waiver.

4. **Time-Limited Waivers and Equivalencies.** An organization can use this tab to request a time-limited waiver to seek additional time (beyond the 60 days required in the ESC) to address an EC or LS Requirement for Improvement (RFI) or SPFI. This request must be made within 30 days from the end of survey. Time-limited waivers are for deficiencies that can be tied to the *Life Safety Code* and/or Health Care Facilities Code.

WHY DO I NEED TO KNOW THIS NOW?

The complexity of the *Life Safety Code* reflects the complexity, scope, and severity of potential risks. As an accreditation professional, you'll need to be involved in the development and management of the SOC, among other documentation required for LS compliance, so getting a handle on this area now is important.

WHERE DO I START?

- **Collaborate with experts.** Work closely with life safety (and environment of care) experts, clinical experts, vendors, and the local fire department on fire drills, fire response plans, *Life Safety Code* assessments, and fire safety equipment inspection, testing, and maintenance compliance.
- **Learn more.** Attend educational programs to learn about fire and life safety issues (and commonly used terms such as fire rating of the wall assembly) and share best practices with other organizations like yours. Books and other resources are also available.
- **Provide education.** Help staff understand the concept of smoke compartments and where they start and end. For example, how can you tell the difference between a door and a smoke or fire door in your organization? When surveyors are on site, they use life safety drawings to confirm where compartments begin and end. Staff ability to identify smoke compartments and knowing how to evacuate horizontally are common findings during survey.
- **Lead training.** Train staff on your fire response plan, including use of a fire response method such as RACE (**R**escue, **A**larm, **C**ontain, **E**vacuate/**E**xtinguish) and a fire extinguisher method such as PASS (**P**ull pin, **A**im nozzle, **S**queeze trigger handle, **S**weep the base of the fire from side to side). You may use a different approach when training students, volunteers, and licensed practitioners. For example, at and away from the fire's point of origin and preparing for building evacuation, students, volunteers, and licensed practitioners follow staff instructions to ensure their safety. This means a nursing student precepting on the unit would be directed by nursing staff to close doors, and licensed practitioners would be asked to help move care recipients to the next smoke compartment.
- **Conduct building assessments.** Perform frequent *Life Safety Code* building assessments to identify risks and to be ready for survey, including documentation that building systems have been tested and are functional.

KEY CONCEPT

ASSESSING RISKS

One or more members of staff must be made responsible for compliance with the *Life Safety Code*, including assessing the facility for compliance with the code, maintaining the BBI, and resolving any code compliance problems. Assessing fire and life safety risks is a critical element of this job. Fire and life safety risks can be identified in several ways, including through testing and inspection activities, optional environmental tours or required fire drills, and preconstruction risk assessments (PCRAs). Reach out to staff in each department. They will be familiar with the specific fire and life safety hazards in their work areas.

Assessment Opportunities

There are several methods for assessing fire risks. The four primary methods described in the following list approach fire safety and life safety from both environmental and process-related perspectives.

1. **Environmental tours.** Although not required by The Joint Commission, environmental tours can be used to assess fire safety and life safety in your organization. Frequencies are defined by the organization.
2. **Construction assessment.** A critical component of any construction project, a PCRA is required by Standard EC.02.06.05, EP 2. PCRAs address the impact of construction or maintenance projects on care and treatment for individuals, as well as occupant safety, before construction begins. In addition, EC and LS standards require organizations to assess, manage, and act to minimize fire safety risks throughout the life cycle of any demolition, construction, or renovation projects. (See "Interim Life Safety Measures" for more information.)
3. **General maintenance and testing.** No matter the size of your organization, you have some fire equipment and fire safety building features that require general maintenance and testing. The frequency of maintenance and testing will vary based on the equipment and/or features your organization uses.
4. **Fire drills.** Fire drills are both a practice exercise for responding to fire events and a method to assess the effectiveness of your fire response plan.

WHY DO I NEED TO KNOW THIS NOW?

Many aspects of the physical environment will be managed by facilities directors and/or safety/security directors. However, you can facilitate risk assessment activities such as fire drills and environmental tours.

WHERE DO I START?

- **Work with experts.** Facilities directors and safety/security directors will take the lead to ensure that the physical environment is safe in your organization. Work with these directors to ensure that all required risk assessments are being conducted and documented.
- **Take a tour.** You don't need to participate in a formal environmental tour to assess the physical environment. If your organization struggles with certain

fire safety or life safety standards, walk through the facility occasionally to see performance improvement activities or note areas that need to improve.

- **Document.** Documentation can be paper or electronic, but make sure all risk assessments are documented in accordance with Joint Commission standards.

KEY CONCEPT

INTERIM LIFE SAFETY MEASURES

Life Safety Code deficiencies cannot always be resolved immediately. Also, construction, maintenance, and repair activities can temporarily compromise the facility's code compliance. In these cases, special safety measures, known as interim life safety measures (ILSMs), must be applied to help ensure the safety of care recipients, staff, visitors, vendors, contractors, and others in the building. ILSMs can include extra fire drills, signage indicating alternate exits, fire watches, environmental rounds, and other activities designed to mitigate risks associated with construction or prolonged noncompliance.

Develop a Policy

All accredited programs aside from laboratories and office-based surgery practices are required to develop a policy to cover the institution of any needed ILSM. It is recommended that behavioral health care and human services organizations also develop such a policy. The policy should detail which ILSMs are appropriate to a given deficiency or construction project, based on the scope and location of the deficiency or project.

Get the Word Out

Any time you institute ILSMs in a given area of the facility, you need to inform staff of the special conditions through signage, message boards, intranet sites, and other applicable means. Be careful not to overcomplicate ILSMs for staff. For example, the lead time to order a new door is six weeks because of a two-inch undercut issue. More than likely most staff, including nurses, will not change their response to a fire or smoke event. As such, select your ILSM based on the issue and impact on staff.

WHY DO I NEED TO KNOW THIS NOW?

Construction, renovation, and general repairs can cause upset in any health care setting. You need to know what measures have been implemented to address any compliance-related issues that may arise.

WHERE DO I START?

- **Work with the team.** Most large-scale construction or renovation projects will be conducted by a team with members from inside and outside the organization. Work with this team to ensure that your organization's ILSM policy is being followed.
- **Know the policy.** Make sure you are aware of what steps need to be taken to ensure that *Life Safety Code* deficiencies that occur because of construction-related or general maintenance activities are resolved.

"I heard that...

if a surveyor discovers an Immediate Threat to Health or Safety, we will be denied accreditation."

fact:

You will, if it's your initial survey. However, if you are being resurveyed and a situation is deemed an Immediate Threat to Health or Safety (also known as "Immediate Threat to Life" or ITL), it will prompt a Preliminary Denial of Accreditation, and you have 72 hours to remedy the situation or risk losing accreditation. If more time is required to fully eliminate the ITL, an abatement survey is conducted within 23 days. In the environment of care, failure to maintain the following five critical facilities systems may trigger an ITL condition: a compromised (1) fire alarm system, (2) sprinkler system, (3) emergency power supply system, (4) medical gas master panel, or (5) exit. Of course, other situations outside the environment of care can trigger an ITL too. Organizations should regularly check systems to ensure that any issues are being addressed effectively, including whether the appropriate interim life safety measures or mitigation actions are in place.

CRITICAL CHALLENGES

Every year The Joint Commission publishes a list of standards that surveyors scored most often in the previous year. The list is broken down for each type of accreditation program, but many of these standards highlight issues that are challenging for all organizations. A review of the trends in these data shows two standards that might be challenging as you address fire safety and life safety in your organization.

CHALLENGING LIFE SAFETY STANDARDS

Fire safety and life safety are critical components for any health care organization. An organization must maintain open paths of egress (LS.02.01.20) and ensure that fire extinguishing systems are in working order (LS.02.01.35) for the safety of everyone in its facility.

What's the problem? Ensuring that care recipients, staff, and visitors can safely exit a facility should not be in question. Many facilities just don't have adequate storage space for all the medical equipment commonly in use today, and staff end up leaving it in hallways.

Many organizations struggle to keep hallways clear of clutter, thus being noncompliant with Standard LS.02.01.20.

For fire extinguishing systems, typically, the problems are in the sprinkler details, such as the following:

- Computer cables resting on or affixed to sprinkler pipes
- Sprinkler heads rusted or painted over
- Not enough clearance around the sprinklers in storage spaces

Standard LS.02.01.35—which requires organizations to provide and maintain fire extinguishing systems—continues to be a deficiency that organizations have trouble complying with.

WHY DO I NEED TO KNOW THIS NOW?

As an accreditation professional, you should be aware of what compliance challenges your organization struggles with.

WHERE DO I START?

- **Review recent risk assessments and survey reports.** Review any past survey reports to see where your organization struggled with its most recent survey. You also can review recent risk assessments to identify where performance improvement activities may be needed to bring fire safety and/or life safety equipment and features into compliance.

EQUIVALENCIES

Equivalencies are an option to address *Life Safety Code* deficiencies that cannot be immediately fixed. Typically, they are used during construction or when other difficult-to-meet conditions are present that cannot be immediately corrected. There are two types of equivalencies:

1. A Traditional Equivalency is a request to maintain building features that are not compliant with the adopted edition of the *Life Safety Code* (NFPA 101).
2. Developed by the NFPA, a Fire Safety Evaluation System (FSES) equivalency objectively deducts specific values for building deficiencies from the building's overall numerical value. (The FSES is a grading system used to evaluate the overall level of a building's fire safety, applying a numerical value as the sum of a building's features.)

For organizations that **do not** use The Joint Commission for deemed status, an equivalency is a Joint Commission–approved alternate approach to address a *Life Safety Code* deficiency.

For deemed status. For organizations that use Joint Commission accreditation for CMS deemed status, CMS must approve all LS and EC time-limited waivers and equivalencies for hospitals and critical access hospitals via the regional office.

TOOLS

Sprinkler System Compliance Checklist

Testing by Time Frame Checklist

Test Your Knowledge

1. Using Joint Commission requirements, indicate whether each item is related to fire safety or life safety.

Fire drills	☐ Fire safety	☐ Life safety
Automatic sprinkler suppression system	☐ Fire safety	☐ Life safety
Fire-rated doors and doorway	☐ Fire safety	☐ Life safety
RACE and PASS	☐ Fire safety	☐ Life safety

2. The Centers for Medicare & Medicaid Services' Conditions of Participation (CoPs) are aligned with which year's edition of the National Fire Protection Association's *Health Care Facilities Code*?
   - ☐ a. 2000
   - ☐ b. 2012
   - ☐ c. 2018
   - ☐ d. 2022

3. Which of the following are examples where interim life safety measures need to be put in place? (Select all that apply.)
   - ☐ a. Egress corridor blocked due to construction
   - ☐ b. Fire alarm panel shut down for maintenance
   - ☐ c. Fire drill
   - ☐ d. Temporarily converting an office into a triage station

---

* *Life Safety Code*® is a registered trademark of the National Fire Protection Association, Quincy, MA.

Infection Prevention and Control

CHAPTER 13

THE BIG IDEA

In health care organizations, implementing infection prevention and control (IC) practices is critical to ensure the health and safety of individuals receiving care, treatment, and services, as well as staff, providers, and visitors. This applies to all health care settings, including outpatient and residential settings. Because the threat is pervasive, the response must be comprehensive: Protection against infection requires an intensive interdisciplinary effort and must always be practiced everywhere within the organization. Please note that the IC chapter on E-dition and in the *Comprehensive Accreditation Manuals* is currently in the process of being revised. The primary concepts remain the same, however.

KEY CONCEPTS

- Infection Prevention and Control Program and Plan
- Transmission of Infections
- Managing IC in the EC

THE MANUAL

Following are the relevant Joint Commission E-dition® or *Comprehensive Accreditation Manual* chapters:

- "Care, Treatment, and Services" (CTS) [behavioral health care and human services only]
- "Environment of Care" (EC)
- "Human Resources" (HR) [not behavioral health care and human services]
- "Human Resources Management" (HRM) [behavioral health care and human services only]
- "Infection Prevention and Control" (IC)
- "Leadership" (LD)
- "National Patient Safety Goals" (NPSG)
- "Performance Improvement" (PI)
- "Provision of Care, Treatment, and Services" (PC) [not behavioral health care and human services or laboratory]

KEY CONCEPT

INFECTION PREVENTION AND CONTROL PROGRAM AND PLAN

The IC program must be managed by an appointed person with clinical expertise in IC or access to IC experts. This individual could be, for example, an infection preventionist or a clinical leader with training and/or expertise in IC, such as an infectious disease practitioner, a public health liaison, a consultant, or another professional with an applicable health care background. The IC program manager must have the knowledge and, preferably, expertise in the relevant issues, as they are responsible for the daily management of all IC activities. Those activities must be done according to a written IC plan. Please note that an appointed person and an IC plan are not required for every accreditation setting. Consult the appropriate *Comprehensive Accreditation Manual* or its E-dition counterpart to ensure that your organization is complying with the right standards.

Infection Prevention and Control Program

Joint Commission standards specify required components of the IC program, including the following:

- **Risks identified by analyzing components.** Risks are identified and prioritized by analyzing each component of the organization (including all locations) that make up the organization and the care, treatment, and services that each provides:
  - Its geographic location, community, and population served
  - The care, treatment, and services it provides
  - The analysis of surveillance activities and other infection control data
- **Goals based on risks.** The plan includes goals based on identified and prioritized risks, typically done via annual risk assessments. Activities (or interventions) are designed to meet those goals. Goals may include how to secure the necessary resources for activities and how to communicate responsibilities for the following:
  - Addressing prioritized risks
  - Limiting unprotected exposure to pathogens
  - Limiting the transmission of infections associated with procedures
  - Limiting the transmission of infections associated with the use of medical equipment, devices, and supplies
  - Improving compliance with hand hygiene guidelines
- **Evaluation based on data.** The plan is reviewed using relevant data at least annually to determine if its goals have been met. The IC plan contains a written description of surveillance activities and evaluates the goals and implementation of IC activities that were identified in the IC plan. High-quality surveillance data include both process measures/performance measures and outcome measures. (*See* Chapters 7 and 8 for more on your role in working with data.) These surveillance data are reported to the organization staff and leadership team and may be reported to external authorities.

PICTURE THIS

Hierarchy for Creating Your Organization's Infection Prevention and Control (IC) Processes, Policies, and Procedures

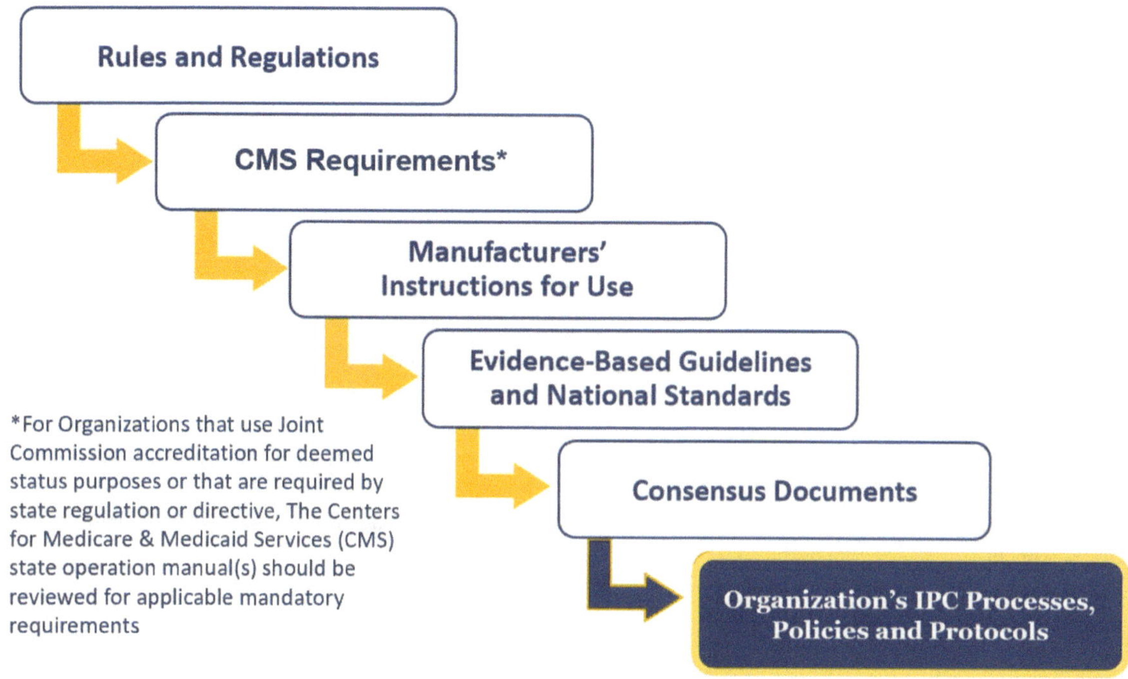

* For organizations that use Joint Commission accreditation for deemed status purposes or that are required by state regulation or directive, Conditions of Participation (CoPs) and/or Conditions for Coverage (CfCs) should be reviewed for applicable mandatory requirements.

Joint Commission standards and elements of performance (EPs) are designed to allow each individual health care organization to determine the best methods and practices for its facility. The Joint Commission, however, is finding that many organizations build policies on evidence-based guidelines alone, believing they will meet the requirements of Joint Commission Infection Prevention and Control (IC) standards and EPs.

IC requirements vary across the United States because of different state and local regulations, devices and equipment, and care practices. The Joint Commission's Leadership (LD) standards require that organizations adhere to applicable federal, state, and local regulations and laws. The Joint Commission recommends that health care organizations (when creating or revising IC-related policies) apply the hierarchical methodology displayed here to address the various IC requirements relevant to the organization. This graphic illustrates the hierarchy of various references that organizations should use as resources when they draft and/or revise their IC-related policies. Not all references will have information that an organization needs to include in its policies, but all required references should be incorporated into processes for use.

WHY DO I NEED TO KNOW THIS NOW?

Organizations should ensure that they have IC activities, including surveillance, to minimize, reduce, or eliminate the risk of infection. IC activities should address the risks/goals identified and pertain to care, treatment, services, and populations served. It is critical that organizations review standards and EPs to ensure that all requirements are captured, including transmission-based precautions and adherence to US Centers for Disease Control and Prevention (CDC) standard precautions.

Top Challenging Infection Prevention and Control Standards

These IC standards and EPs are those that have recently been most frequently cited by Joint Commission surveyors as being non-compliant.

Standard	Element of Performance (EP)	Applicable Accreditation Program(s)
IC.02.01.01: The organization implements the infection prevention and control activities it has planned.	**EP 1:** The organization implements its infection prevention and control activities, including surveillance, to minimize, reduce, or eliminate the risk of infection.	Home Care
IC.02.01.01: The organization implements the infection prevention and control activities it has planned.	**EP 2:** The organization uses standard precautions, including the use of personal protective equipment, to reduce the risk of infection.	Ambulatory Care, Home Care, Nursing Care Center, Office-Based Surgery
IC.02.02.01: The organization reduces the risk of infections associated with medical equipment, devices, and supplies.	**EP 1:** The organization implements infection prevention and control activities when doing the following: Cleaning and performing disinfection of medical supplies and devices.	Ambulatory Care, Home Care
IC.02.02.01: The organization reduces the risk of infections associated with medical equipment, devices, and supplies.	**EP 2:** The organization implements infection prevention and control activities when doing the following: Performing intermediate and high-level disinfection and sterilization of medical equipment, devices, and supplies.	Ambulatory Care, Critical Access Hospital, Hospital, Office-Based Surgery
IC.02.02.01: The organization reduces the risk of infections associated with medical equipment, devices, and supplies.	**EP 4:** The organization implements infection prevention and control activities when doing the following: Storing medical equipment, devices, and supplies.	Hospital, Nursing Care Center

TOOL

Infection Prevention and Control Plan Assessment Checklist

WHERE DO I START?

- **Collaborate with experts.** Serve on your organization's IC committee, if appropriate for your organization. Connect with your organization's infection preventionist, if applicable, and other IC staff.
- **Review documents.** Review the IC plan with the IC program manager and make sure it includes all requirements from the standards, including annual risk assessments. Make a point to be part of any evaluations and updates of the plan.
- **Work with leaders.** Set up regular meetings with leaders—including clinical leaders—about the IC program budget to avoid logistical logjams when your program needs funds.
- **Work with data.** Review infection-related surveillance data to make sure results of IC plan activities align with the IC plan goals. You also may want to look at how data relate to mortality reports, customer complaint reports, sentinel events, and what IC data or issues are reported to QAPI.

KEY CONCEPT

TRANSMISSION OF INFECTIONS

All health care facilities are responsible for preventing the transmission of infections to care recipients, staff, providers, and visitors. This means implementation of activities and interventions to break the cycle of infection transmission. After developing an IC plan and activities with this goal in mind, you must implement it. This includes ensuring that health care workers are trained in the IC policies/procedures specific to the facility and their roles.

PICTURE THIS

Proactive Infection Prevention and Control (IC) Risk Assessment Cycle

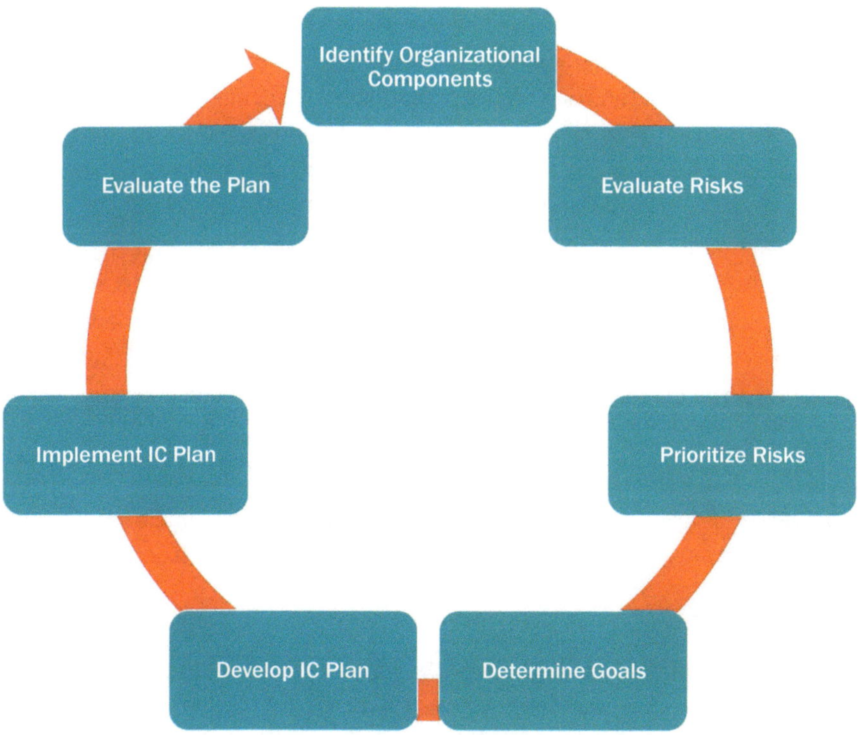

Identify Organizational Components
Evaluate Risks
Prioritize Risks
Determine Goals
Develop IC Plan
Implement IC Plan
Evaluate the Plan

Risk assessment is the cornerstone of any good IC program. As this diagram illustrates, infection prevention and control (IC) risk assessments include many steps that are outlined like a road map in the standards. As you conduct IC risk assessments in your organization, it is important to involve leaders and other key staff when necessary. This diagram shows the circular nature of continuous improvement each year.

Vulnerable Populations

Some organizations have particularly vulnerable populations, such as the following:

- **Hospitals,** which have neonatal and pediatric wards, burn units, and bone marrow transplant programs
- **Nursing care centers and assisted living communities,** which have elderly care recipients who are particularly susceptible to infections
- **Home care agencies,** which typically have care recipients with specific conditions, such as wounds, compromised immune systems, urinary catheters, and vascular catheters and ports, as well as individuals undergoing dialysis

Particular care must be taken to keep vulnerable populations safe from infection transmission risks.

Types of Precautions

The following types of precautions are implemented to prevent the transmission of infectious agents:

- **Standard precautions.** Implemented across the organization, these precautions are used to protect against possible exposure to infections and include measures derived from the Core Infection Prevention and Control Practices of the CDC, such as hand hygiene, safe use and disposal of sharps, and correct use of personal protective equipment (PPE). Standard precautions also include maintaining a clean environment with the cleaning, disinfecting, and sterilizing (CDS) of medical equipment, devices, and supplies, including the reprocessing of reusable medical devices.
- **Transmission-based precautions.** Implemented for individuals with contagious pathogens or who are potentially contagious, these precautions typically involve implementing activities aimed at preventing the transmission of certain infectious organisms and may include patient placement (single patient room, for example) and using appropriate PPE. They may also involve ventilation methods to prevent the spread of airborne infections. Implementation of transmission-based precautions may differ depending on the setting (for example, inpatient, outpatient, long-term care), the facility design characteristics, and the type of interaction with the individual. The implementation should be adapted based on the health care setting.

Staff Vaccinations

Staff vaccination can be important to protect them from occupational exposure, decrease the severity of illness, and protect those they provide care for and work with.

Positive outcomes. Achieving and sustaining high vaccination rates among health care workers, specifically influenza vaccinations, can lead to positive health outcomes, such as the following:

- Reducing the transmission of viruses to other staff, care recipients, and families
- Decreasing morbidity and mortality rates among care recipients
- Reducing medical expenses and workforce absenteeism
- Ensuring preparedness for possible pandemics

PICTURE THIS

The Chain of Infection

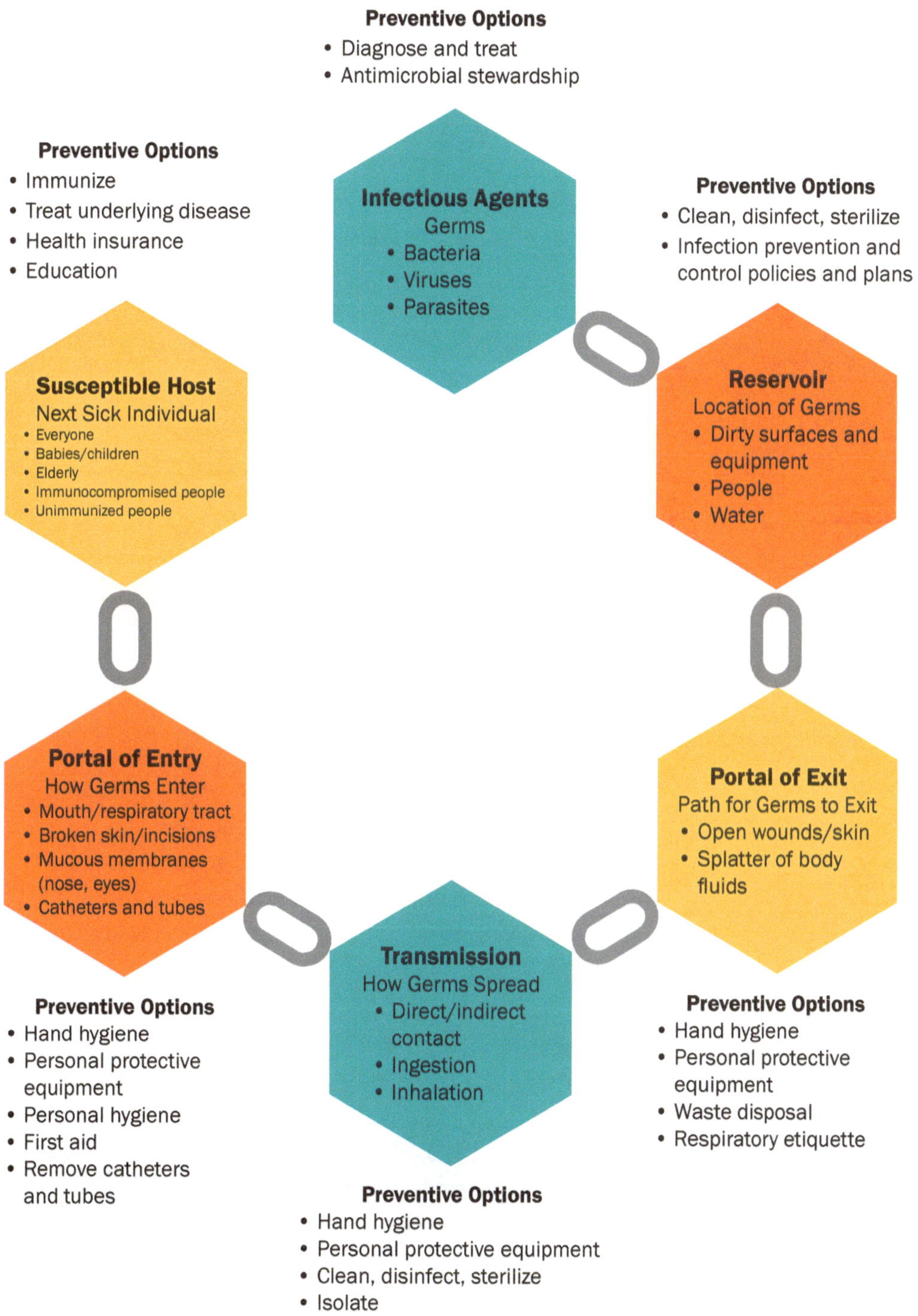

The chain of infection is the path that an infection follows to propagate itself. This illustration shows the path to infection with examples of what propagates each chain. In addition, the checkmarked list shows potential actions to take to break the chain. It is critical to have a comprehensive IC program to block the transmission of infectious agents.

"I heard that...

The Joint Commission requires health care organizations to fire staff who don't get an annual flu shot."

fact:

Although The Joint Commission requires organizations to offer influenza vaccinations to licensed practitioners and staff, it doesn't require them to face termination if they choose not to be vaccinated. The Joint Commission also doesn't require accredited organizations to pay for their organization's staff to receive flu shots.

TOOL

Staff Immunization Assessment Checklist

Timely Response to Emerging Threats

Microorganisms can cause epidemics, pandemics, or infectious disease outbreaks, or be used in acts of bioterrorism. Infection can spread quickly without strategic readiness and sufficient resources to manage an influx of individuals needing care. That's why The Joint Commission requires you to have a written plan to address an influx of potentially infectious care recipients. (One acceptable response is to not accept individuals needing care.)

WHY DO I NEED TO KNOW THIS NOW?

Influenza, coronavirus, and other infectious diseases can become epidemics or, as we recently experienced, pandemics. You must make sure your organization is prepared for an epidemic, or you could be overwhelmed in a crisis.

WHERE DO I START?

- **Conduct tracers.** Participate in or lead targeted tracers to check that protocols for clinical decision support are being followed in various areas of your organization (for example, central processing, housekeeping, surgery, endoscopy).
- **Review documents.** Read your organization's plan for infectious disease emergencies. Check also to make sure IC is included in emergency management (EM) policies and exercises and participate in the EM exercises. (See Chapter 10 for more information about emergency management.)

KEY CONCEPT

MANAGING IC IN THE EC

An important intersection occurs between IC and the environment of care (EC), also known as the physical environment of a health care organization. Several environmental factors can affect infection rates—from the materials used to construct facilities to the number and placement of sharps disposal containers. Environmental cleaning and care of equipment, furniture, and other surfaces, as well as replacing worn or damaged items, also have an impact. This connection is evident in cross-references between the IC and EC standards.

Medical Equipment

Medical equipment and devices need to be clean and functioning correctly during use to keep patients safe and avoid risk of infection. But what about when they aren't in use? For example, it is crucial that flexible endoscopes be safe for use for care recipients. All staff involved in reprocessing this equipment must understand and consistently follow several standardized steps to ensure that all scopes are reprocessed appropriately. As the body of knowledge about reprocessing procedures and technology is always growing, it is essential that IC programs and procedures are regularly reviewed to ensure that they are following manufacturers' instructions for use as well as local, state, regional, and federal rules and regulations.

Depending on your setting of care, you may be working with EC staff as well as biomedical engineers, central processing staff, infection preventionists, and housekeeping to address these IC needs. During emergencies or disasters, that collaboration is intensified.

Utilities

Utility systems, such as air handling, ventilation, heating, and water distribution systems, can both prevent and pose infection risks. For example, negative pressure rooms can prevent airborne infectious agents from spreading. Drinking fountains, ice machines, and other equipment that contains or uses water pose risks for spreading waterborne pathogens (including *Legionella*), unless properly maintained. Utility systems therefore need to be designed and maintained to support IC activities. For example, organizations should have a water management program to define the necessary maintenance tasks and to assign staff responsibilities to prevent infection risk. Hospitals, critical access hospitals, and nursing care centers accredited by The Joint Commission must have a water management program that addresses *Legionella* and other waterborne pathogens. These programs must be in accordance with law and regulation.

Hazardous Waste

Simple tasks such as taking out the trash require heightened attention to detail. Infectious/medical waste (also known as regulated medical waste, biohazard waste, and biomedical waste) require proper handling to prevent spread of infection when it's generated, when it's labeled, when it's transported, and when it's disposed of.

Construction

Planning, designing, constructing, and renovating new and existing health facilities can be an exciting task, but it can also lead to potential infection. That's why The Joint Commission requires organizations to include IC in its planning and design of areas or building to be renovated or constructed, in addition to the requirement to conduct an infection control risk assessment (ICRA) before starting any construction activity to ensure that care recipients, visitors, and staff are protected from exposure to dust, which could contain pathogenic mold.

Environmental Cleaning and Disinfection

Contaminated surfaces contribute to the transmission of pathogens, which can survive and remain pathogenic for long periods of time.

To ensure that environmental surfaces are safe and comply with Joint Commission Standard EC.02.06.01, your organization must devise clearly defined cleaning and disinfection policies and procedures and ensure compliance with environmental services and housekeeping protocols for surfaces. These surfaces commonly include floors, walls, furnishings, sinks, carpets, and curtains.

To do this, your organization must determine which cleaners and disinfectants to use and how they should be used (and when making these decisions, you should rely on evidence-based information). In addition, your environmental services team will need to develop policies and protocols that include the following:

- Selecting cleaners and disinfectants, and trialing and evaluating them
- Using cleaners and disinfectants properly
- Training staff and testing competency for using cleaners and disinfectants
- Monitoring cleaning and disinfection practices, and evaluating them
- Ensuring a standardization of products across departments
- Evaluating new technologies to assist with environmental hygiene
- Approving new products through a multidisciplinary organizational committee
- Using appropriate tools and products for cleaning and disinfecting

Many types of cleaners and disinfectants are available, and they are continuously evolving.

WHY DO I NEED TO KNOW THIS NOW?

If you learn the basics of the IC/EC connection now, you can work with the IC/EC experts to imagine the worst situations and aim for the best practices to prevent them. (See Chapter 11 for more about the environment of care.)

WHERE DO I START?

Note: *In some organizations, particularly larger ones, many IC tasks are performed by infection preventionists or facility managers, not accreditation professionals.*

- **Know the requirements.** Refer to state regulations related to infection prevention and control to better understand the requirements.
- **Review documents.** Read your organization's policies and procedures for hazardous waste management to see how they deal with infectious/medical waste.
- **Collaborate with experts.** Work with facility engineers, environmental services, and IC experts to provide a clean, safe, functional environment and to decrease the risk for transmission of infectious agents.

CRITICAL CHALLENGES

Every year The Joint Commission publishes a list of standards that surveyors scored most often in the previous year. The list is broken down for each type of accreditation program, but many of these standards highlight issues that are challenging for all organizations. A review of the trends in these data shows two areas of focus that might be challenging as you address infection prevention and control in your organization.

HAND HYGIENE

Hand hygiene is the #1 best practice for infection prevention and control. All care recipients, staff, families, and visitors should follow good hand hygiene practices before and after all encounters with care recipients and certain clinical interventions.

What's the problem? Standard IC.01.04.01, Element of Performance (EP) 1, requires that organizations have a goal for compliance with hand hygiene guidelines based on their risk assessment. (And NPSG.07.01.01 requires that organizations improve performance toward that goal.) Compliance challenges include educating staff, care recipients, families, and visitors and ensuring that everyone is provided with facilities and opportunities to practice good hand hygiene and to monitor and continually improve efforts for staff and care recipient compliance.

Supporting Hand Hygiene Practice

You probably know this: Health care workers don't always follow hand hygiene protocols. But you may not know this: Studies show a need for continuing staff education about the importance of this simple yet critical safeguard. Other factors that have a positive impact on hand hygiene performance include the following:

- Leadership support
- Friendly reminders
- Not adding to staff workload
- Convenient availability of products
- Integrating the protocols into routine procedures
- Enhanced monitoring of systems as they relate to hand hygiene

PI and a Hand Hygiene Program

A hand hygiene program is required, in accordance with NPSG.07.01.01. Compliance with this goal is an ongoing performance improvement (PI) activity in many organizations (as mentioned previously, improving compliance is a required goal in the IC plan). Surveyors typically ask to see hand hygiene PI data.

WHY DO I NEED TO KNOW THIS NOW?

If you can get staff, care recipients, providers (including licensed practitioners), and visitors to improve compliance with hand hygiene, you'll see a significant decrease in morbidity and mortality among individuals receiving care due to infection. You'll also be helping to protect everyone from acquiring infections.

WHERE DO I START?

- **Conduct tracers.** Work with the IC program manager to plan or lead frequent hand hygiene tracers. Make this a part of IC surveillance activities.
- **Review documents.** Make sure your organization's hand hygiene program documents specify which hand hygiene guidelines you're using. You're required to use either the CDC's and/or the World Health Organization's guidelines.
- **Work with data and leaders.** After reviewing your organization's data on hand hygiene compliance, meet with organization leaders, PI leaders, and infection preventionists about your hand hygiene program. Discuss the possible need for new approaches.
- **Involve frontline staff.** Frontline staff may have unique insights into how programs are applied and what makes them successful. Provide opportunities for frontline staff to propose hand hygiene and other IC program solutions.
- **Provide education.** Work with your communications department and infection preventionists to develop staff, provider, and care recipient education materials (such as posters, videos, buttons, and stickers) that address barriers to hand hygiene compliance.

TOOL

Physical Environment Hand Hygiene Assessment Checklist

HIGH-LEVEL DISINFECTION

High-level disinfection (HLD) of medical/surgical devices helps reduce the spread of infection. The CDC has created a classification for the high-level disinfection of devices such as respiratory therapy equipment and endoscopes, which due to their usage can acquire microorganisms that may cause infection. Other guidelines for HLD have been released by the Society of Gastroenterology Nurses and Associates (SGNA), the Association for the Advancement of Medical Instrumentation® (AAMI), and other professional organizations.

What's the problem? Compliance with **IC.02.02.01, EP 2,** can be challenging, given the complexity of some devices and how often the devices are used.

- **Lack of familiarity.** All staff involved in the disinfection and sterilization of devices and equipment must be familiar with the Spaulding Classification, which classifies devices and instruments according to the disinfection and sterilization practice that's required. They must know how an item will be used to confirm that the appropriate Spaulding Classification is followed.

- **Lack of education.** All staff who perform sterilization must also be trained in the specifics of sterilization, low-level disinfection, and HLD procedures, including such concepts as the flow of instruments or devices from dirty to clean, maintenance and quality monitoring of equipment and devices used in the process, and use of adjunct supplies in accordance with manufacturer's instructions for use and proper storage practices.

WHY DO I NEED TO KNOW THIS NOW?

Reducing the spread of infection is a critical reason proper HLD procedures must be followed.

WHERE DO I START?

- **Educate.** Make sure staff in charge of HLD know the specifics of sterilization, low-level disinfection, and HLD procedures. Also ensure that staff are familiar with the Spalding Classification

Test Your Knowledge

1. According to Joint Commission requirements, which of the following are key components of an infection prevention and control plan? (Select all that apply.)
   - ☐ a. Annual evaluation of data
   - ☐ b. Establishment of goals
   - ☐ c. Risk assessment
   - ☐ d. Annual budget
2. When an organization is creating its policy for instrument reprocessing, which source of guidance should it NOT consider?
   - ☐ a. Law and regulations
   - ☐ b. Media coverage of an infectious disease outbreak involving that instrument
   - ☐ c. Manufacturer's instructions for use for that instrument
   - ☐ d. Evidence-based guidelines
3. Which of the following are types of proactive risk assessments? (Select all that apply.)
   - ☐ a. Infection control risk assessment
   - ☐ b. Failure mode and effects analysis
   - ☐ c. Preconstruction risk assessment
   - ☐ d. Hazard vulnerability assessment
4. Which infection prevention and control issues are considered high risk from a Joint Commission viewpoint?
   - ☐ a. Influenza vaccination
   - ☐ b. Instrument processing
   - ☐ c. Hand hygiene compliance
   - ☐ d. Proper wearing of personal protective equipment
5. Which of the following disciplines need to work closely with your infection prevention and control practitioner? (Select all that apply.)
   - ☐ a. Governing body and communications
   - ☐ b. Medical staff and clinical lab
   - ☐ c. Pharmacy and clinical staff
   - ☐ d. Leadership and supply chain

Leadership

CHAPTER 14

THE BIG IDEA

Leaders—individual leaders and groups of leaders—in a health care organization work collaboratively to set expectations, develop plans, and improve the quality of the organization's governance and management as well as its clinical and support functions and processes. To carry out this responsibility, leaders use the mission, vision, and goals of the organization to guide them.

KEY CONCEPTS

- Leadership Structure and Responsibilities
- Role in Performance Improvement
- Safety Culture
- Operations and Change Management

THE MANUAL

Following are the relevant Joint Commission E-dition® or *Comprehensive Accreditation Manual* chapters:

- "Leadership" (LD)
- "Patient Safety Systems" (PS) [not assisted living community or behavioral health care and human services]
- "Safety Systems for Individuals Served" (SSIS) [behavioral health care and human services only]

KEY CONCEPT

LEADERSHIP STRUCTURE AND RESPONSIBILITIES

How leadership is structured differs by organization, but Joint Commission standards require a defined structure. The standards also require defined leadership responsibilities. Leaders in a health care organization include individuals and groups who have varying reporting and collaborative relationships with each other and staff, depending on your organization. This is a typical structure:

- **Governing body.** This group is usually a board of directors or board of trustees (or governance in a military hospital). Its members may or may not have clinical or health care experience.
- **Executive committee.** Although not a requirement, the executive committee is a subgroup of the governing body and is usually made up of officers.
- **Quality committee.** Also not a requirement, this subcommittee of the governing body addresses quality and safety issues, reporting to the full board regularly.
- **Senior managers and leaders.** This group includes executives such as the chief executive officer, nursing home administrator, chief medical officer, chief financial officer, and nurse executive, as well as clinical leaders, and other staff members in leadership positions.
- **Organized medical staff.** This group (present in hospitals and critical access hospitals only) is made up of doctors of medicine and osteopathy and may include other practitioners. They're accountable to the governing body.

Leadership Responsibilities

As a whole, leaders have ultimate responsibility for everything that happens in a health care organization. They're charged with managing the following important functions:

- Sharing the organization's mission, vision, and goals and modeling its values and principles
- Maintaining an environment in which safety is the top priority
- Planning and providing services that meet care recipient needs
- Ensuring resources for care, treatment, and services
- Providing competent staff and other care providers
- Improving performance of functions and processes (*see* Chapter 16 for more about performance improvement [PI])
- Establishing expectations for the performance of contractors and contracted services and communicating them to contractors (see "Critical Challenges" on page 172 for more about compliance challenges in this area)
- Reviewing and approving documentation required by Joint Commission standards

Responsibilities specific to accreditation. It's nearly impossible to achieve and maintain Joint Commission accreditation without the support of leaders.

TOOLS

Governing Board Responsibilities Checklist

Board Quality and Safety Committee Sample Agenda

Top Challenging Leadership Standards

These standards and elements of performance (EPs) are those that have recently been most frequently cited by Joint Commission surveyors for non-compliance.

Standard	Element of Performance (EP)	Applicable Accreditation Program(s)
LD.01.03.01: Governance is ultimately accountable for the safety and quality of care, treatment, or services.	**EP 12: For home health agencies and hospices that elect to use The Joint Commission deemed status option:** The organization has a governing body that assumes full legal authority and responsibility for the overall operation of the organization. **For home health agencies that elect to use The Joint Commission deemed status option:** Overall operation of the organization includes provision of services, fiscal operations, review of the agency's budget and operational plans, and its quality assessment and performance improvement (QAPI) program. **For hospices that elect to use The Joint Commission deemed status option:** A qualified administrator appointed by and reporting to the governing body is responsible for the day-to-day operations of the hospice.	Home Care
LD.04.01.05: The organization effectively manages its programs, services, or sites.	**EP 4:** Staff are held accountable for their responsibilities.	Ambulatory Care
LD.04.05.07: The laboratory director, technical consultant, and/ or technical supervisor are responsible for maintaining laboratory performance.	**EP 4:** The laboratory director, technical consultant, and/or technical supervisor do the following: • Ascertain that the laboratory is enrolled and successfully participates in an approved proficiency testing program that is relevant for each test performed • Review quality control and proficiency testing data • Require corrective action and documentation on unacceptable quality control and proficiency testing results • Evaluate the test results that appear inconsistent with clinically relevant criteria • Discuss with staff any issues that have been identified	Laboratory

Organization leaders must provide resources, of course, but also visible and verbal support, so staff know that it's a priority.

WHY DO I NEED TO KNOW THIS NOW?

Having leadership support for the accreditation process from the very start will make nearly all of your efforts go more smoothly.

WHERE DO I START?

- **Learn more.** The mission and vision of your organization are the foundation for all leadership activities. Find out more about it: How does the organization plan to meet the needs of its population(s)? By what ethical standards does it operate? What does it want to accomplish through its work? Be sure to also review the free board education portal on The Joint Commission's website.

Governing Body and Required Oversight of QAPI Program

The Quality Assessment Performance Improvement (QAPI) CMS Condition of Participation and related Interpretive Guidance found at 42 CFR 482.21 require hospitals to maintain and demonstrate evidence that a hospital's governing body provide oversight of their QAPI program to provide safe, quality patient care and prevent adverse events and patient harm. Hospital leaders play an integral role in advancing the development and sustainment of the QAPI program with active engagement from the hospital's governing body.

The governing body is responsible for oversight of the QAPI program through periodic reviews of the program, which include development of a plan to implement and maintain the program; determine annual QAPI projects; review progress of QAPI projects; and evaluate the effectiveness of improvement actions that have been implemented throughout the hospital. The governing body must also establish and communicate clear expectations for hospital-wide safety and allocate adequate resources to the QAPI program.

TOOL

Proactive Risk Assessment Worksheet

KEY CONCEPT

ROLE IN PERFORMANCE IMPROVEMENT

The Joint Commission holds leaders accountable for all safety and quality functions and processes and for related PI efforts. That's because leaders are the drivers of the organization's mission, vision, and goals, which are typically aimed at the best care possible.

Identifying and Prioritizing Areas of Improvement

All PI activities should be data driven, per the standards. LD standards require leaders to identify and prioritize areas for improvement. Common ways to do that include proactive risk assessments, which can help uncover potential problems, and a comprehensive systematic analysis (such as a root cause analysis), which can help discover the source of a safety problem that has already occurred. Both can give direction in planning process improvements. (*See* Chapter 16 for more on the PI process.)

WHY DO I NEED TO KNOW THIS NOW?

LD standards require an organizationwide, integrated safety program. PI is often part of that. And a PI team simply can't succeed without leadership support and resources. In addition, the LD standards require health care organizations to select one high-risk process and conduct a proactive risk assessment at least every 18 months. You'll probably be involved in that.

WHERE DO I START?

- **Collaborate with experts.** Seek out PI experts in your organization or among your peers. Find out more about how leaders are involved and what tools are being used. Don't be afraid to try new ones.

KEY CONCEPT

SAFETY CULTURE

As you might expect, safety is the top priority in a culture of safety, or a safety culture. But what do we mean by *safety*? There are two meanings here: (1) *safety* for care recipients and staff during clinical and nonclinical activities, and (2) *safety* for staff in reporting errors and sharing information related to safety of care recipients. The basic concept: You can't keep people safe unless everyone feels safe to report problems that threaten safety.

Goals for a Safety Culture

Organizations will have varying levels of safety culture, but all should be working toward a safety culture that has the following qualities:

- **Safety values**. Staff and leaders value transparency, accountability, and mutual respect. Everyone makes safety the first priority.
- **Collective mindfulness.** Staff realize that systems always have the potential to fail and they focus on finding hazardous conditions or close calls at early stages before a care recipient may be harmed. Staff do not view close calls as evidence that the system prevented an error but rather as evidence that the system needs to be further improved to prevent any defects.
- **Reporting culture**. Staff and leaders commit to a safe reporting culture. When system errors occur, they are discussed, and improvement processes are developed to promote a learning environment. Care recipients, staff, and families are encouraged to report unacceptable behaviors that undermine a culture of safety to organization leaders for the purpose of fostering risk reduction. Staff know that their leaders will focus not on blaming providers involved in errors but on the systems issues that contributed to or enabled the patient safety event.

TOOL

Safety Culture Policy Evaluation Checklist

Although not required by The Joint Commission, a Safety Culture Policy can help establish and maintain a safety culture throughout your organization.

Importance of a Safety Culture

A safety culture is the foundation of safety for care recipients and high reliability in your organization. High reliability doesn't just happen by everyone doing their best. It requires a commitment by everyone in the organization, from leaders on down, not only to following safety policies and protocols but also to a constant evaluation and reevaluation of those policies to ensure that they actually work the way they are supposed to.

Developing a Safety Culture

Organization leaders are more than tone setters in this process. Leaders are instrumental in creating the administrative structures that allow for the crucial safety culture activities to take place. Safety culture is built around assessment and PI activities. Therefore, data collection, PI planning, communication, change management, and staffing decisions are all areas where organization leaders can contribute to the development of safety culture.

TOOL

Safety Culture Actions Checklist

Maintaining a Safety Culture

Be transparent and accountable. A safety culture is one in which every employee, regardless of rank or department, feels comfortable reporting safety issues. That comfort level comes from two sources. First, the process of reporting and remedying problems must be as transparent as possible. As with root cause analysis, the focus should be on process improvement, not on individual responsibility. And all staff members should feel that they can be heard and that they know what will happen if they report a safety issue. Second, there must be accountability in the process. Staff won't report problems if they don't believe anything will be done to solve them. A detailed written process for gathering information, trying out fixes, and reporting results of changes to policy or procedure is absolutely essential to giving your employees the sense that they can report problems and help participate in creating solutions.

WHY DO I NEED TO KNOW THIS NOW?

Cooperation for compliance activities requires a culture of safety. Why? In part because changes will likely need to be made, and you—and everyone else—have to feel safe from the start about making changes and reporting problems.

WHERE DO I START?

- **Learn more.** The Joint Commission requires organizations to measure safety culture by using a reliable tool under Standard LD.03.01.01. The Agency for Healthcare Research and Quality (AHRQ) has one such tool, although you can use your own if it's valid and reliable. Also, read the "Patient Safety Systems" (PS)/"Safety Systems for Individuals Served" (SSIS) [behavioral health care and human services only] chapter on E-dition or your setting's *Comprehensive Accreditation Manual*.
- **Review documents.** Look over your organization's related policies and procedures. Is your organization promoting a culture of safety? Is your organization tolerant of bad behavior? Do you need to suggest updating policies and procedures?

PICTURE THIS

Behaviors That Undermine a Culture of Safety

NURSE: Dr. Alma, I need to talk to you about Dr. Dean again. His behavior with the staff is unacceptable. They complain about him every day. He's insulting and uses disrespectful language when he speaks to them.

CMO: Look, he'll be retiring in a few years anyway. Tell your staff to develop a thicker skin.

NURSE: I'm seeing significant stress in my staff due to this situation. I think it's time to talk to the board.

CMO: Bob is an old friend of the chair of our board, Angie. I'd like to help you out, but I think you can handle this. And if you can't, talk to some consultants.

The Joint Commission requires leaders to create and maintain a culture of safety and quality throughout the organization, including managing behaviors that undermine a culture of safety through the use of a code of conduct. Scenarios like this dialogue between a nurse leader and a chief medical officer (CMO) can be used to discuss ways to handle inappropriate behavior, in accordance with your code of conduct.

KEY CONCEPT

OPERATIONS AND CHANGE MANAGEMENT

Decisions made and changes implemented by leaders affect more than just your organization's administration. Day-to-day operations, including care, treatment, and services, can be affected as well. This is why many of the LD standards address operational issues and change management. Here are some examples:

Resources

Making resources—human, financial, and physical—available is one of the key leadership responsibilities cited at the beginning of this chapter. This responsibility includes setting the budget, prioritizing change efforts, hiring sufficient numbers of competent people, and allocating space and equipment within your facilities.

Consider your population(s) of care recipients. Leaders also must consider the organization's specific care recipient populations in resources decisions. For example, are essential supplies available in sizes or amounts appropriate for children and infants? Does your organization have access to translation and interpretation services for those with limited English proficiency? Do your facilities have appropriate access for the disabled according to the Americans with Disabilities Act (ADA) standards?

Similar Care for Similar Issues

It's a time of uncertain and changing health care coverage. Ensuring that care recipients with similar health care issues receive similar care and treatment throughout the organization becomes a focus. Alternate services might be provided depending on an insurance situation or other differences. However, any variances shouldn't significantly affect the outcome of the care provided. That's a Joint Commission LD requirement.

Care Recipient Flow

Problems with care recipient flow result in overcrowding, long waits for admission, and other delays that undermine care. But care recipient flow is usually not an admissions issue—it's a systemwide issue. Every process, from assessment to the cleaning of rooms to discharge, can have an impact on care recipient flow. Leaders must monitor this on a system level.

Conflicts in Ethics and Values

Health care presents a wide range of ethical issues for people and organizations. These values may conflict, often when decisions about treatment are being made. Resolving these issues isn't easy. It must be done in a way that satisfies all parties (to some degree), and that's a challenge for health care leaders. That's where an ethics committee or consultant might be called into play. The people or person in this role should be easily available to all care providers, as well as to other leaders, so they can make the best possible ethical decisions.

WHY DO I NEED TO KNOW THIS NOW?

Every decision leaders make has a potential impact on your compliance efforts. Knowing how they handle operations and change are two key areas to keep an eye on.

WHERE DO I START?

- **Be a bridge.** Help leaders assess the risks by keeping communication lines open with staff about problems. For example, you might organize a regular session for airing issues and soliciting suggestions.
- **Get training.** Change management skills are as essential for accreditation professionals as they are for leaders. Look into training opportunities for these skills in your organization and beyond. Attend training with leaders and build relationships at the same time.

CRITICAL CHALLENGES

Every year The Joint Commission publishes a list of standards that surveyors scored most often in the previous year. The list is broken down for each type of accreditation program, but many of these standards highlight issues that are challenging for all organizations. A review of the trends in these data shows a standard that might be challenging as you address leadership in your organization.

CONTRACTED SERVICES

Nearly all health care organizations use some contracted services, and many find it a challenge to meet standard LD.04.03.09, which relates to that practice: "Care, treatment, and services provided through contractual agreement are provided safely and effectively." (Please note that this standard applies only to contracted services for direct care for care recipients.)

What's the problem? You're dealing with another organization. In addition, challenges may arise due to the services provided and contracts. Although those employees are under contract to your organization, they're not employed by it. In some settings, such as home care, those employees may never even set foot in one of your facilities.

Health care organizations need to establish measurable performance expectations that focus on risk reduction and/or improved outcomes.

Failing to define these expectations leads to leaders failing to monitor the performance of contracted staff based on those expectations.

WHY DO I NEED TO KNOW THIS NOW?

With increasing demands and fewer resources internally, you may find yourself dealing more with contracted services than you expected.

WHERE DO I START?

- **Review documents.** Make sure your list of contracted services is comprehensive and complete.
- **Check documentation.** Are leaders evaluating the organization's contracted services regularly? Are leaders addressing any services that aren't meeting a certain level of quality? Standard LD.04.03.09 requires evaluations but doesn't specify exactly how to conduct them; leaders select a method that best suits the organization. You can help them to do that.
- **Evaluate contracted services.** Ways to evaluate contracted services should be measurable and include the following:
  - Review the contractor's Joint Commission accreditation or certification status.
  - Directly observe the contractor's staff in action.
  - Audit the contractor's documentation, including records of care and credentialing and human resources records, and contracts.
  - Review any incident reports.
  - Have the contracted organization or its individual staffers submit periodic reports.
  - Collect data on the performance expectations, risk reductions, and improved outcomes of the services being provided.
  - Include performance indicators in the contract and monitor those regularly.
  - Get input from staff and the individuals served by your organization.
  - Review satisfaction studies.
  - Review results of risk-management activities.

just imagine...

Care and Treatment with Contracted Services

Your organization's dialysis center, run by a contracted firm, has learned that dialysis equipment is contaminated. During documentation review to discover the source of the contamination, the quality staff finds that the center's medication logs are incomplete. Dialysis staff aren't recording data for each treatment, and no records show that medications have been double-checked before being administered. This makes it difficult to track the contamination and find out which care recipients may have been affected.

Leadership standards require your organization to ensure that care recipients are getting safe and effective care from your contracted services. This means you must monitor their activities and include process measures/performance measures in their contracts. Professional organizations and agencies can provide performance benchmarks.

Test Your Knowledge

1. Which of the following are key components of leadership for a hospital? (Select all that apply.)
   - ☐ a. Staff
   - ☐ b. Governing body
   - ☐ c. Executive management
   - ☐ d. Organized medical staff
2. A staff member observed a potential work hazard, but their coworkers told them not to report it, because it would bring attention to their team. Which of the following are correct statements? (Select all that apply.)
   - ☐ a. This is an example of a culture of safety.
   - ☐ b. Reporting should be done without fear of punishment.
   - ☐ c. Safety culture says, "Report anyway!"
   - ☐ d. Leadership sees these reports as more unnecessary work.
3. During an internal assessment, frontline managers stated that organization leaders intentionally understaff their program to reach financial targets, which they believe has led to patient safety issues. Which of the following statements is correct?
   - ☐ a. Organization leaders have the responsibility to provide resources necessary to meet the organization's mission.
   - ☐ b. The governing body should recommend changing the mission of the organization.
   - ☐ c. Leaders can direct programs according to requirements from the community and stakeholders.
   - ☐ d. A financial audit is required by Joint Commission standards.
4. According to Joint Commission requirements, who is responsible for organizational performance improvement?
   - ☐ a. Executive managers
   - ☐ b. Governing body
   - ☐ c. Medical staff
   - ☐ d. Quality director

Medication Management

CHAPTER 15

THE BIG IDEA

Medication management is composed of a complex system of processes focused on an overall goal of medication safety. Creating and maintaining that system is an interdisciplinary responsibility that involves prescribers, nurses, and pharmacists working with care recipients and their families. It's also a system that often affects several health care settings, so coordination of care related to medications can present many challenges.

KEY CONCEPTS

- Relationship to Other Standards
- Medication Management Processes
- Medication Errors
- Medication Reconciliation
- Medication Orders
- High-Alert and Hazardous Medications

THE MANUAL

Following are the relevant Joint Commission E-dition® or *Comprehensive Accreditation Manual* chapters:

- "Care, Treatment, and Services" (CTS) [behavioral health care and human services only]
- "Environment of Care" (EC)
- "Human Resources (HR) [not behavioral health care and human services]
- "Human Resources Management" (HRM) [behavioral health care and human services only]
- "Infection Prevention and Control" (IC)
- "Information Management" (IM)
- "Leadership" (LD)
- "Medication Management" (MM) [not laboratory]
- "National Patient Safety Goals" (NPSG)
- "Provision of Care, Treatment, and Services" (PC) [not behavioral health care and human services or laboratory]
- "Record of Care, Treatment, and Services" (RC) [not laboratory]
- "Rights and Responsibilities of the Individual" (RI)

KEY CONCEPT

RELATIONSHIP TO OTHER STANDARDS

In the standards on E-dition and in the *Comprehensive Accreditation Manual* "Medication Management" (MM) chapter, you'll notice cross-references to standards in other chapters. They're all related. It happens frequently with MM standards. Here's why:

- **MM and RC (Record of Care, Treatment, and Services).** Medication information must be recorded and updated in the record of care, which is covered by the RC standards.
- **MM and IC (Infection Prevention and Control).** Safe handling and compounding of medications is part of both medication management and infection prevention and control practice. Proper antibiotic stewardship is also part of both medication management and infection prevention and control.
- **MM and IM (Information Management).** Many medical records are stored electronically, which makes them subject to IM standards. A list of prohibited abbreviations for medication documentation and orders is also in the IM chapter. Maintaining the integrity of the record of care and maintaining and adhering to the prohibited abbreviations list are two ways information management contributes to safe medication management. A "Prohibited Abbreviations" list (which includes the ones mentioned in the IM standards) is also provided in Chapter 17 of this book.
- **MM and EC (Environment of Care).** Hazardous medications are disposed of under requirements for disposing of other hazardous materials, as addressed by the EC standards. Recall of medications by federal agencies is also part of the EC team duties.
- **MM and PC (Provision of Care, Treatment, and Services) or CTS (Care, Treatment, and Services).** Emergency medications, as well as new and self-administered medications, require a heightened focus on the care recipient's needs, risks, and education and are the PC and CTS chapters' domain.
- **MM and RI (Rights and Responsibilities of the Individual).** Pain management and investigational medications, which need to comply with standards related to the rights of the individual, are covered in the RI chapter.
- **MM and NPSG (National Patient Safety Goals).** These goals cover many patient safety issues, including those related to safe use of anticoagulants (see NPSG.03.05.01), medication reconciliation (see NPSG.03.06.01), and labeling on and off the sterile field in the operating room and procedure areas (*see* NPSG.03.04.01).
- **MM and LD (Leadership).** Leaders are responsible for creating a culture that prioritizes safety and is conducive to an environment that is supportive of medication error reporting. LD standards also cover contracted services, which may be used for pharmacy or other medication-related services.
- **MM and HR (Human Resources) or HRM (Human Resources Management).** Requirements in the HR[M] chapter cover many staff competency issues as well as education and training. Staff must have specific skills and knowledge to provide competent medication-related care.

WHY DO I NEED TO KNOW THIS NOW?

Medication management is a complex process that is affected by multiple chapters and external processes. These processes must be effective and compliant to ensure the safety of individuals receiving care, treatment, and services. When you understand the relationship between standards across chapters, you're in a better position to provide complementary compliance strategies for those standards.

WHERE DO I START?

- **Facilitate processes.** Become familiar with standards cross-referenced in the MM chapter. Look for incomplete compliance or noncompliance trends among related standards to identify larger system issues. Consider interdisciplinary meetings on sets of related standards to discuss complementary processes and approaches.

KEY CONCEPT

MEDICATION MANAGEMENT PROCESSES

A medication management system is made up of interactive processes that flow across a health care organization. These processes may include the following:

- Planning
- Selection and procurement
- Storing (and securing)
- Ordering (prescribing and transcribing)
- Preparing
- Dispensing
- Administration
- Monitoring
- Evaluation

MM System Tracers

The MM requirements address all processes in a medication management system. (In fact, the first MM standard, MM.01.01.01, is about planning those processes.) Joint Commission surveyors often conduct medication management system tracers. System tracers reveal problems with system issues and care recipient issues (see Chapter 4 for more information about system and individual tracers).

Adaptable Policies

These processes can be very difficult to manage in some organizations. For example, in home care and large health care systems, the wide range of health care settings pose particular challenges. Creating adaptable policies (based on size, population served, and so on)—and implementing them consistently—takes careful planning.

Top Challenging Medication Management Standards

The following Medication Management standards and elements of performance (EPs) are those that have recently been frequently cited by Joint Commission surveyors for non-compliance.

Standard	Element of Performance (EP)	Applicable Accreditation Program(s)
MM.01.01.03: The organization safely manages high-alert and hazardous medications	**EP 2:** The organization follows a process for managing high-alert and hazardous medications.	Ambulatory Care, Office-Based Surgery
MM.01.02.01: The organization addresses the safe use of look-alike/ sound-alike medication.	**EP 2:** The organization takes action to avoid errors involving the interchange of medications on its list of look-alike/sound-alike medication.	Ambulatory Care, Office-Based Surgery
MM.06.01.01: The organization safely administers medications.	**EP 3:** Before administration, the individual administering the medication does the following: • Verifies that the medication selected matches the medication order and product label • Visually inspects the medication for particulates, discoloration, or other loss of integrity • Verifies that the medication has not expired • Verifies that no contraindications exist • Verifies that the medication is being administered at the proper time, in the prescribed dose, and by the correct route • Discusses any unresolved concerns about the medication with the patient's licensed practitioner, prescriber (if different from the licensed practitioner), and/or staff involved with the patient's care, treatment, and services	Critical Access Hospital, Hospital

WHY DO I NEED TO KNOW THIS NOW?

Getting to know your medication management system will help you identify opportunities to improve medication safety and will prepare you for these types of tracers during survey.

TOOL

Medication Management System Stakeholder Analysis Form

WHERE DO I START?

- **Work with staff.** Meet with key staff in each part of your medication management system to get a sense of compliance hot spots. Refer to the MM standards and your organization's related policies and procedures. Make sure to account for all parts of your organization; include how any off-site medication practices are integrated into your system.

KEY CONCEPT

MEDICATION ERRORS

To err is human—and common. But system faults may be at the root of the most common causes of medication errors. According to the US Food and Drug Administration (FDA), the most common causes of medication errors are the following:

- Poor communication (incomplete patient information, miscommunication of medication orders)
- Confusion in product names, dosing units, and medical abbreviations
- Incorrect labeling
- Care recipient's misunderstanding directions for medication use

Look-Alike/Sound-Alike Medications

Many medications have names that look or sound like the names of other medications. Organizations must keep a list of such medications and create a

PICTURE THIS

Look-Alike/Sound-Alike Drug Dangers

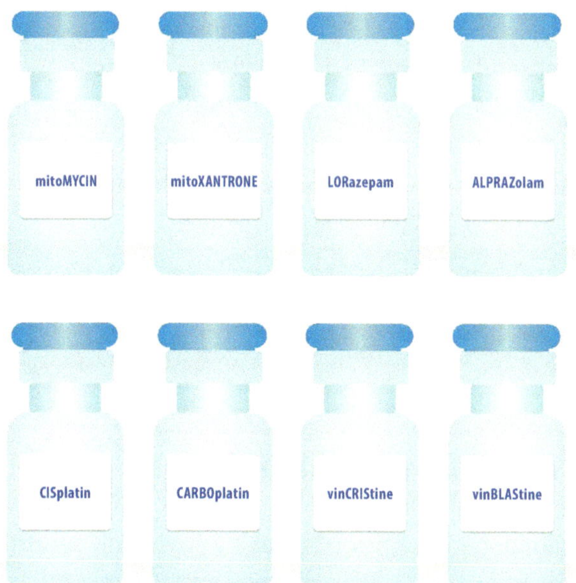

A 2014 *International Journal of Clinical Pharmacy* study estimated that 25% of medication errors were due to look-alike/sound-alike medication (LASA) pairs. Some LASA pairs are chemotherapy drugs classed as both high-alert and hazardous medications. Tall-man lettering on labels, like those shown above, can be very helpful in distinguishing these pairs.

TOOL

Look-Alike/Sound-Alike Medication Management Policy Development Checklist

policy to help avoid confusion and medication errors. The list must be reviewed and updated at least annually in accordance with Joint Commission standards.

Reporting Medication Errors

In accordance with Standard MM.07.01.03, Element of Performance (EP) 3, and organizationwide policy, all staff are required to report actual or potential adverse drug events (ADEs), significant adverse drug reactions (ADRs), and any medication errors. Staff and providers who are blamed for errors may be less inclined to report them. Lack of reporting such errors leads to more risk, particularly if the incidents actually have roots in system issues. Respecting those who report errors is part of a culture of safety (see Chapter 14).

TOOL

Medication Error Investigation Procedure Checklist

For deemed status. The US Centers for Medicare & Medicaid Services (CMS) expects immediate notice to take place when harm to a patient has already occurred due to a medication error or where there is potential for harm as a result of the medication error. If the outcome of the error is unknown, the physician must also be notified immediately, as addressing the needs of the patient must be the priority.

WHY DO I NEED TO KNOW THIS NOW?

Knowing the most common causes of medication errors may help you focus on contributing factors within your organization. Awareness of the impact of blame in reporting errors can help to empower employees to report incidents without fear of retribution. Both knowing and maintaining awareness should be on your awareness radar as you head toward survey (that is, always).

WHERE DO I START?

- **Provide education.** All providers, prescribers, and staff should be aware of when and how to report medication errors, according to your organization's policy. Provide in-service training on this topic frequently to make sure everyone is clear about what to do when mistakes occur.
- **Work with data.** Look at incident reports to see how errors are being categorized. Do they provide meaningful data to use for improvement efforts (see Chapter 16 for additional information on performance improvement activities)? How else might data be collected?

just imagine...

Multidose Vial Use

While at the care recipient's bedside, a nurse inserts a needle into a multidose vial (MDV) and administers the medication to the recipient. Because there is medication left in the vial, he returns it to the medication cart. He later uses the same vial of medication on another care recipient, thus introducing a potential infection to the second recipient.

MDVs should be dedicated to a single care recipient whenever possible. If MDVs must be used for more than one care recipient, they should not be kept or accessed in the immediate treatment area. This is to prevent inadvertent contamination of the vial through direct or indirect

(continued)

KEY CONCEPT

MEDICATION RECONCILIATION

Medication reconciliation is about maintaining and communicating accurate medication information. It's a process that involves many people working together, which can result in varying perspectives and may lead to challenges in agreement. Medication reconciliation should happen, at a minimum, at the beginning and end of an episode of care.

PICTURE THIS

Admission Medication Reconciliation

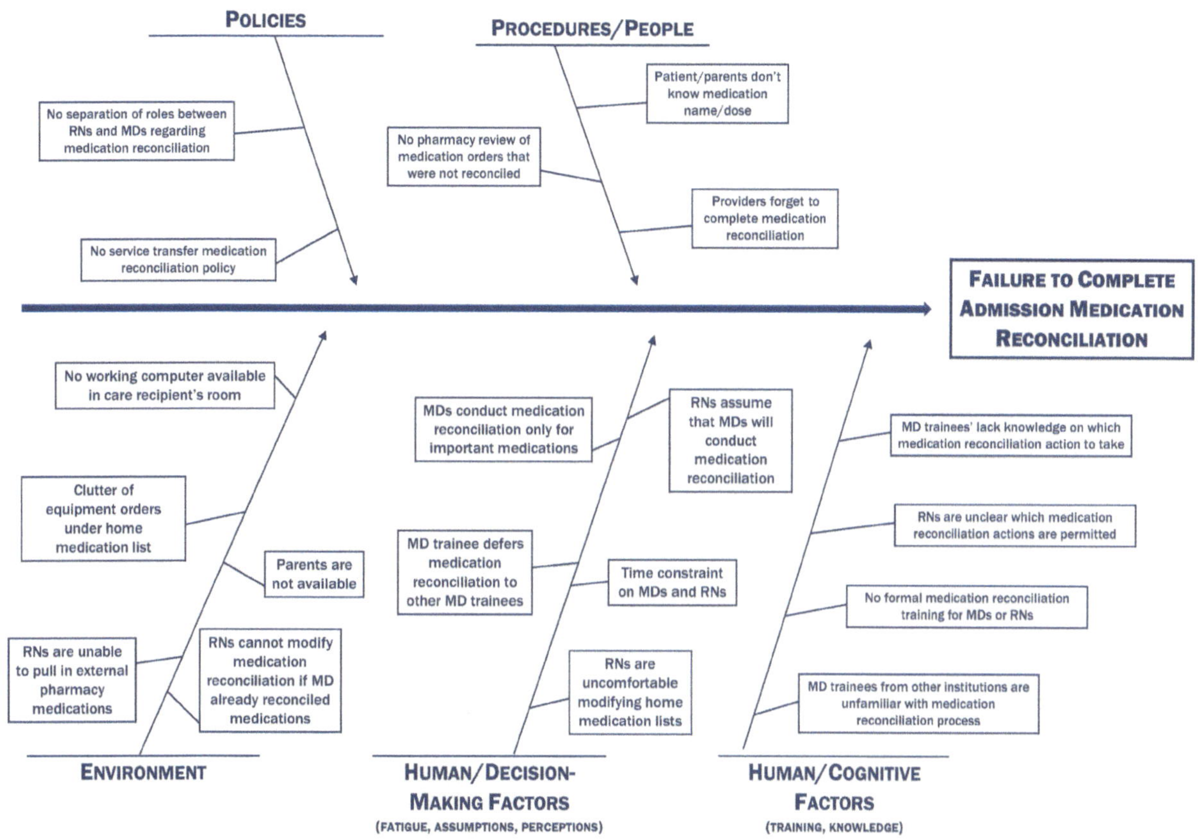

This fishbone diagram illustrates several important factors that can contribute to medication reconciliation problems and errors.

At Admission and Discharge

Most medication reconciliation happens at admission and discharge or whenever new medications are ordered. Given the scope of clinical condition of care recipients, obtaining their medication information can be challenging. The Joint Commission recognizes a good faith effort to collect this information as meeting the intent of the requirement.

Care recipient and family medication education. When medications are prescribed, you must do more when you're giving medication information to care recipients (and their families) at discharge. Standard PC.02.03.01, EP 10, requires organizations to provide information and education on the safe and effective use of medications. NPSG.03.06.01 requires you to provide the following:

- Written information about the medications the patient or individual should be taking
- Education about how to manage the patient's or individual's medication information (such as maintaining a current list of medications)

(continued)

contact with potentially contaminated surfaces or equipment that could then lead to infection in subsequent care recipients. If an MDV enters the immediate treatment area of a care recipient, it should be dedicated to that individual only and discarded after use. Examples of the immediate treatment areas include care recipient rooms or bays and operating rooms. When a medication is accessed in a direct care area, the vials are considered single use and are discarded upon completion of that care recipient's case.

WHY DO I NEED TO KNOW THIS NOW?

The care recipient and family are an integral part of the medication management system. The sooner you get comfortable with involving them in your compliance efforts, the better.

WHERE DO I START?

- **Provide education.** Does staff in-service training for medication reconciliation address the patient-facing requirements? Encourage staff to practice with volunteer care recipients and families in an effort to reinforce the use of a medication card.

just imagine...

Medication Education for Self-Administered Medications

A care recipient discharged from the hospital began taking four 1 mg tablets of warfarin daily. A week later, after a fall, he was readmitted, and the warfarin was increased to 6 mg daily. At discharge, a new prescription was written for 6 mg tablets. No one at the hospital instructed the care recipient or his wife about the new dosage or that he should take only one pill daily rather than four times a day. Five days later, the wife called the home health nurse to ask a question; the nurse visited that day to perform a care assessment. She discovered that the wife had been giving her husband four 6 mg tablets daily—24 mg daily instead of the prescribed 6 mg daily. The care recipient was admitted to intensive care until the danger passed.

Care recipient and family education about medications, is vital during transitions of care. This is particularly important with self-administered medications, which are common in home care, nursing care centers, ambulatory care, and behavioral health care and human services.

KEY CONCEPT

MEDICATION ORDERS

A large percentage of medication errors occur when new orders are written during the admission or discharge of a care recipient. Of course, incomplete, illegible, or unclear orders at any point along the care continuum can lead to medication errors. That's why all medication orders must be clear and accurate—wherever and whenever medications are ordered, dispensed, and administered. The idea is to curtail confusion to eliminate errors.

Typical Pitfalls

Confusion in medication orders often arises from PRN (as needed) indicators and dose range orders with unclear parameters. Verbal orders can cause confusion too, so for most organizations, qualified individuals must authenticate any verbal medication order with read-back for verification. Verbal orders (including telephone orders) should be kept to a minimum, and texting orders are prohibited. (See Chapter 17 for additional information on verbal orders.)

WHY DO I NEED TO KNOW THIS NOW?

Knowing reasons for errors helps you focus your monitoring lens. Also, medication ordering standards are aimed at prescribers, who may not be employed by your organization. If they are not familiar with Joint Commission standards, you may need to monitor them closely as well.

WHERE DO I START?

- **Review documents.** Review your organization policy on medication orders and make sure it includes everything required by the MM standards. Consider adding needed requirements from the standards into your policy as well as specifics on how range orders should be interpreted.
- **Conduct tracers.** Perform regular audits of medication orders as part of your mock tracers to assess for sustained compliance.
- **Provide education.** Along with the audits, educate staff on how to respond to noncompliant medication orders per your policy. You might want to provide them with a brief script they could use when calling prescribers to clarify an order.

- **Facilitate processes.** Review preprinted orders and order sets to ensure that they support safe prescribing. Work with staff and providers to get ideas on how they can be improved.
- **Encourage technology use.** Required elements of medication orders can be built into a computerized provider order entry (CPOE) system for increased assurance.

KEY CONCEPT

HIGH-ALERT AND HAZARDOUS MEDICATIONS

It's common to think of all medications as beneficial—and that's certainly the intent. But in addition to possible side effects and other ADRs, some medications are dangerous if not handled correctly.

High-Alert Medications

High-alert medications, such as epinephrine and insulin, are drugs that bear a heightened risk of causing significant harm to care recipients when they are used in error. High-alert medications require special attention because the consequences of an error with these drugs are clearly more devastating to the care recipient. The Institute for Safe Medication Practices (ISMP) has resources with lists of high-alert medications by setting (see "Recommended Resources" near the end of this book for links). Your organization should develop your own list addressing medications used in the organization.

Hazardous Medications

Medications are considered hazardous because unprotected exposure to them can cause serious harm—to care recipients, visitors, providers, and staff. Cytotoxic drugs used in chemotherapy are an example of a hazardous medication. Because these drugs can become part of the physical environment via spills and leaks, The Joint Commission also discusses them (in addition to Standard MM.01.01.03) in the EC chapter's hazardous materials and waste standard, EC.02.02.01, EP 8. (See Chapter 11 for more about hazardous materials.)

WHY DO I NEED TO KNOW THIS NOW?

When anything is termed *high-alert* or *hazardous*, you need to know about it as soon as possible, and this includes staff, who may require extra training on handling these highly dangerous drugs.

WHERE DO I START?

- **Collaborate with experts.** Schedule regular meetings with pharmacists to keep up to date on the required formulary lists for high-alert medications and hazardous medications stocked by your organization. Talk about the processes to mitigate risks within each category. Work with environment of care staff on disposal of any hazardous medications.
- **Provide education.** Pull together high-alert and hazardous medications resources available from ISMP, the US Occupational Safety and Health

"I heard that...

The Joint Commission says you have to cancel all medication orders and then rewrite them all when a patient moves from one level of care to another."

fact:

Joint Commission standards require that patient information, such as medication orders, travel with the patient and that care, treatment, and services be provided using the most recent patient orders. Your organization, however, may develop a policy that goes beyond Joint Commission requirements. In that case, surveyors will survey your organization to the strictest requirements, even if they're your requirements.

Administration (OSHA), and the National Institute for Occupational Safety and Health (NIOSH). Make them available in one place for all staff to reference.

- **Conduct tracers.** Make high-alert and hazardous medications a periodic focus for tracers in relevant areas of your organization.

CRITICAL CHALLENGES

Every year The Joint Commission publishes a list of standards that surveyors scored most often in the previous year. The list is broken down for each type of accreditation program, but many of these standards highlight issues that are challenging across all health care organizations. A review of the trends in these data shows three standards that might be challenging as you address medication management in your organization.

ANTIBIOTIC STEWARDSHIP

According to the US Centers for Disease Control and Prevention (CDC), there are at least 2.8 million antibiotic-resistant infections each year. Optimizing the use of antibiotics is a patient safety priority, and antibiotic stewardship programs play a critical role in supporting appropriate prescribing and reducing antibiotic resistance.

What's the problem? Medication Management (MM) Standard MM.09.01.01 (for hospitals, critical access hospitals, and nursing care centers) or Standard MM.09.01.03 (for ambulatory care organizations) requires organizations to have an antibiotic stewardship program to help curb the excessive or inappropriate use of antibiotics.

- **Elements of an antibiotic stewardship program:**
  - **Commitment.** Leaders bear the responsibility of providing financial resources to support the antibiotic stewardship program, appointing a leader of the program, and outlining responsibilities. Leaders also must support the program in less tangible ways, making it clear that the program is an organizational priority. For example, leaders can be vocal in backing and recognizing the efforts of those contributing to the antibiotic stewardship program.
  - **Accountability.** Data and results from the program must be reported to appropriate individuals and committees, including care recipient safety staff, infection prevention and control experts, and senior leaders.
  - **Multidisciplinary scope.** Within your organization you should bring together pharmacists, infectious disease physicians, infection prevention and control professionals, and

microbiologists to oversee the antibiotic stewardship program. Working with the guidance of outside experts, such as those at the CDC and other public health and professional organizations, you can get the best information and practices into the hands of those who may be overprescribing antibiotics and help to manage departments with dangerously high levels of antibiotic use.

- **Measurement.** What you measure and how you measure it will determine the quality of your antibiotic stewardship program. Good data help you understand if and how current practices at your organization may be creating resistance and identify opportunities for improvement. Furthermore, you will need to be able to track your efforts at reducing resistance. Data scientists can help. Also, the Agency for Healthcare Research and Quality (AHRQ) has created tools and resources to help organizations like yours generate meaningful data about your antibiotic stewardship program's efficacy.
- **Education.** New protocols and trends in antibiotic resistance must be communicated to clinical staff, through formal education events and other internal methods of communication. This will give your frontline staff the tools and best practices they need to achieve the program's goals.

WHY DO I NEED TO KNOW THIS NOW?

Antibiotics are necessary medications used to treat specific infections. When overprescribed or incorrectly prescribed, antibiotics are not effective.

WHERE DO I START?

- **Reference the Joint Commission Antibiotic Stewardship Resources.** This portal provides information to support organizations across health care settings in their efforts to improve antibiotic stewardship and decrease antibiotic resistance. It can be accessed on The Joint Commission's website.
- **Establish or sustain an antibiotic stewardship program.** If a program does not exist in your organization, reach out to leaders and infection preventionists in your organization to create an antibiotic stewardship program. Emphasize that this is a required program to remain compliant with Joint Commission standards. If you are working in an organization that has an established antibiotic stewardship program, become involved to support the program and ensure continued compliance.

MEDICATION STORAGE

What's been the top challenging MM standard across all health care organizations in recent years? Standard MM.03.01.01: Safely store medications.

“I heard that...

The Joint Commission requires meds to be secured in a two-lock system.”

fact:

The Joint Commission doesn’t require a two-lock system for any medications (although your state may). And it only requires locking up of controlled substances. All other medications can be kept in secure, unlocked spaces (such as a med room or operating room) if authorized individuals identified in the organization policy control access to the area.

TOOL

Medication Storage and Security Assessment Checklist

What’s the problem? This standard is challenging because it involves two hard-to-control factors:

- **The human factor.** The time and effort to secure drugs means that staff sometimes forget or neglect to do it.
- **The environmental factor.** Many medications must be stored under specific temperature and humidity conditions. If a drug isn’t stored under the correct conditions, it’s not safe to use. Home care organizations often face unique challenges. What if the home isn’t clean or doesn’t have consistent temperature control or adequate refrigeration? In that case, another storage location might be needed.

WHY DO I NEED TO KNOW THIS NOW?

When one standard keeps showing up across all types of organizations as a challenge, pay attention to it. It could spell trouble for your organization as the standard has in others. Also, knowing about these hard-to-control factors will help you evaluate medication storage compliance strategies better.

WHERE DO I START?

- **Organize information.** Get familiar with the general topics covered by the many medication storage EPs, looking for how problems in your organization line up with these EP topics:
  - Ensuring appropriate conditions for medication storage
  - Securing controlled substances
  - Requiring policies for handling, storing, securing, and returning medications from provision/dispensing by the pharmacy until administering to the care recipient
  - Labeling stored medications
  - Inspecting medication areas
  - Handling expired medications
  - Incorporating sample medications in your plans, if your organization uses these

DRUG DIVERSION

The US Substance Abuse and Mental Health Services Administration and the American Nurses Association estimate that 10% of health care workers abuse drugs. The availability and access to medications in health care organizations makes it difficult to detect and prevent drug diversion.

What’s the problem? Controlled (scheduled) medications are used in a variety of health care contexts. It can be challenging to keep these medications secure (in accordance with Standard MM.03.01.01, EP 3) and track them in all types of situations (in accordance with MM.05.01.11, EP 2).

- Keeping all medications and biologicals, including controlled (scheduled) medications, secure is required. Keeping controlled substances locked is required when necessary, in accordance with law and regulation (to prevent drug diversion). In home care and community-based behavioral health care and human services, secure options for medication storage may vary depending on the setting. Therefore, advice from a local pharmacist can be helpful. In ambulatory care centers, safe storage of sample medications is an increasing concern.

WHY DO I NEED TO KNOW THIS NOW?

Stricter control of medications and prescribing has been associated with rising rates of diversion. Health care and health care support professionals have some of the proportionally highest rates of death due to natural and semisynthetic opioids, according to recent CDC data.

WHERE DO I START?

- Create a strong antidiversion system that tracks all controlled (scheduled) medications.
- Ensure that all staff are following the policy.
- Institute appropriate controls on automated dispensing machines.
- Invest in technology-based recordkeeping and tracking systems.

Test Your Knowledge

1. Medication errors always cause patient harm.
   - ☐ a. True
   - ☐ b. False
2. Which of the following statements about adverse drug events is correct?
   - ☐ a. The event is considered an adverse drug event only if the patient gets admitted to an emergency department or intensive care unit.
   - ☐ b. An adverse drug event can be expected or unexpected.
   - ☐ c. An adverse drug event requires reversal agents.
3. Which of the following statements about medication reconciliation is correct?
   - ☐ a. Except for the Laboratory and Point-of-Care Testing Accreditation program, all other accreditation programs have a medication reconciliation requirement.
   - ☐ b. Medication reconciliation is done once (at the point of entry into an organization).
   - ☐ c. The medication reconciliation requirement has staff members reviewing the patient's medication at every encounter.
   - ☐ d. Medication reconciliation is dependent on a pharmacist's oversight.

Performance Improvement

CHAPTER 16

THE BIG IDEA

Performance improvement (PI) is not simply collecting data. It's a systematic and continual process of using data to monitor and understand organizational performance. It involves collecting data, analyzing those data to identify improvement opportunities, and implementing interventions. It also involves monitoring and adapting the interventions based on further collected data and sustaining any improvements resulting from the interventions. These efforts are so important in health care that many organizations have their own PI departments and specialists.

KEY CONCEPTS

- Performance Improvement Approaches
- Improvement Infrastructure
- Improvement Team
- Improvement Opportunities
- Improvement Recognition

THE MANUAL

Following are the relevant Joint Commission E-dition® or *Comprehensive Accreditation Manual* chapters:

- "Leadership" (LD)
- "Performance Improvement" (PI)

KEY CONCEPT

PERFORMANCE IMPROVEMENT APPROACHES

The Joint Commission doesn't mandate which type of methodology that health care organizations use, but they do need to use some PI methodology consistently. Among the most common models used by PI professionals are the PDSA (**P**lan-**Do**-**S**tudy-**A**ct) or PDCA (**P**lan-**Do**-**C**heck-**A**ct), the Toyota Production System, and Six Sigma's DMAIC (**D**efine, **M**easure, **A**nalyze, **I**mprove, **C**ontrol). Several approaches created specifically for PI have been used successfully across health care settings.

Goal of Performance Improvement

The goal of PI is simple and nearly always the same: to make a function or a process better. There are as many methods to assess and implement PI ideas as there are PI goals to achieve. PI has a few basic steps that will be similar no matter the project, but the tools, team, scope, complexity, and so on will vary for each project. Initiating, leading, or participating in PI processes for your organization will lead to some of the more rewarding moments as an accreditation professional.

Basic Steps of the PI Process

You cannot improve a process or function if you can't identify key components that may need to be assessed. Assessing the data gathered will lead to the final step of improving. To ensure the validity and sustainability of the improvements, these steps are usually repeated. The following three steps are the foundation for all PI projects:

1. **Measure.** Collect valid, reliable data on a function or process—data about how the function/process is working. Such data may become part of an internal database.
2. **Assess.** Analyze collected data and translate information. The information is used to draw conclusions about performance, identify improvement opportunities, and set priorities for those improvement opportunities.
3. **Improve.** Develop, test, and implement certain changes (interventions), either by redesigning an existing process or designing a new one. Define objectives for how the intervention will improve performance.

Sustaining Improvements

Don't underestimate the importance of a sustainability plan. Your team should incorporate one into your approach—one that includes an ongoing monitoring system, as well as a plan of what to do if the improvements start to slip.

FMEA and Root Cause Analysis

The Assess step of the PI process often involves benchmarking, a comprehensive systematic analysis (such as a root cause analysis [RCA]), and sometimes tools such as failure mode and effects analysis (FMEA). FMEA and RCA differ in critical ways but also share similarities.

Differences. The fundamental difference between the two tools is timing. RCA is a retrospective approach, whereas FMEA is a proactive approach, designed to keep unwanted events from occurring in the first place. In other words, RCA asks "Why?" after an event has occurred to identify the root causes of the event; FMEA asks "What if?" to explore what could happen if a failure occurred at a specific step in a process.

Similarities. FMEA and RCA have the following characteristics in common:

- They're both nonstatistical methods of analysis.
- The goal of both is to reduce the possibility of future harm to care recipients.
- They both involve identifying conditions that lead to harm.
- They're both team activities.

Interconnections. As methodologies, FMEA and RCA can be—and often are—interconnected. FMEA can be used during an RCA to help evaluate various improvement strategies that resulted from RCA. FMEA can look at where the various strategies might fail and identify any new failure modes that have been introduced as a result of new design processes. RCA can be used to identify the root causes of failure modes.

Reassessment

As you work your way through any intervention approach, be sure to reassess your priorities as necessary. The first improvement intervention you try might not work, and that's okay. Just go back and try something else.

WHY DO I NEED TO KNOW THIS NOW?

Having a grasp of the basic steps in PI is a fundamental part of your job. PI is typically one of the more rewarding components of an accreditation professional's work. You must know how it works to help it work. If you don't understand the basic processes to create change and improve performance, you'll find it hard to know when and how to measure the success of your efforts—and you must measure them to meet various Joint Commission standards.

WHERE DO I START?

- **Review documents.** Look at the documentation of previous or ongoing PI efforts to get a sense of how your organization approaches the three basic PI steps. Ask questions of your improvement team, if one exists: Who is involved at each step? Where are the data stored?
- **Facilitate processes.** Work through each step of your action plan in a thoughtful, methodical fashion. Don't rush. And identify appropriate measures to help define and track improvement.

TOOLS

Design Failure Mode and Effects Analysis (DFMEA) Template

Root Cause Analysis Evaluation Checklist

UNDERSTANDING FIRST-ORDER AND SECOND-ORDER CHANGE

The only constant in life is change. Organization staff and leaders must be proactive in their assessments of how the organization, or their unit, functions so that the organization can implement PI projects before problems become critical.

Leadership (LD) Standard LD.03.05.01 requires leaders to manage change, with an emphasis on quality and safety. Through the effective use of data collection and analysis, planning, communication, changing performance, and effective management of staffing, leaders can react to the myriad changes that confront the organization. However, this is not merely a reactive process. Leaders should consider proactive PI activities that are fundamental or systemic in nature, called second-order change.

First-order change. First-order changes are more limited, reactive changes to policy or procedure that are meant to remedy identified deficiencies and return a system to its proper functioning. Reeducation is a commonly used method of first-order change.

Second-order change. Second-order changes are more sweeping in nature. They seek to substantially improve the functioning or efficiency of the whole system or large parts of it. They aim to produce improvement in many different areas by multiple measure. When you implement second-order change, you are fundamentally changing the way that process works to achieve a better outcome.

Organization leaders must avoid getting caught up reacting to first-order change management, though these activities are important. In a sense, leadership lies in the ability and willingness to take a more holistic approach to improvement. Second-order change is

(continued)

KEY CONCEPT

IMPROVEMENT INFRASTRUCTURE

PI should be built into every aspect of your organization, at every level. That's why it's critical to understand the PI infrastructure that's in place or prepare to develop a clearly defined infrastructure if it doesn't exist.

PI starts at the top. Leaders at all levels set priorities for PI. Leaders are also responsible for involving a broad array of staff and care recipients in PI activities. And it is ultimately up to leaders to implement and manage change initiatives identified by the PI team. Ultimately, it's the leaders who have responsibility for PI. They decide which improvement goals have priority and allocate resources accordingly. (See Chapter 14 for more on leadership responsibilities.)

Executive Leadership Level

- **Who are they?** Typically, this includes the board of directors, as well as the chief executive officer (CEO) or administrator, chief operating officer (COO), chief medical officer (CMO), chief nursing officer (CNO), and chief quality officer (CQO).
- **What do they do?**
  - Set strategic imperatives
  - Provide resources
  - Heighten awareness of PI needs and expectations throughout the organization
  - Hold senior leaders accountable for PI activities in their departments

Senior Leadership Level

- **Who are they?** Examples of individuals at this level include department chairs, medical and nursing directors, facility directors, quality directors, and accreditation and regulatory professionals.
- **What do they do?**
  - Coordinate the strategic imperatives set at the executive level
  - Analyze the current capacity to lead and spread PI
  - Define how to reach the goals and delegate resources
  - Monitor, respond to, and share PI reports
  - Hold frontline leaders and staff accountable for PI initiatives

Frontline Leadership Level

- **Who are they?** This group may include attending physicians, clinical nurse specialists and other clinical leaders, mid-level providers, staff nurses, care recipient managers, and pharmacists.
- **What do they do?**
  - Decide how to integrate PI interventions into clinical practice
  - Monitor effects of interventions
  - Evaluate the functionality of interventions

- Provide education and rapid feedback on interventions to frontline staff
- Make reports about interventions at regular meetings

WHY DO I NEED TO KNOW THIS NOW?

The chain of command is the basis for accountability, reliability, and trust. For PI, it sets the tone of cooperation and teamwork that's necessary for improving performance throughout the organization.

WHERE DO I START?

- **Organize information.** Create a comprehensive organizational chart that clearly shows the reporting structure, naming leaders at all levels. Update it as needed and share it at periodic PI meetings as a reminder of who is accountable for what.

a challenge to manage because it affects so many more people, requires much more material commitment, and takes longer to achieve. But second-order change is essential to health care organizations' ability to evolve to meet new environmental and regulatory challenges, meet changing community health care needs, and advance the cause of safety and high reliability.

KEY CONCEPT

IMPROVEMENT TEAM

Your ability to help improve performance will depend heavily on the improvement team(s). Whether one exists already or you assemble one, the best teams have a sufficient number of people with a variety of perspectives and the right mix of skills to fill different roles. It's important to include some members of the frontline staff (such as nurses), as they are typically the most involved in the PI activity.

Team Roles

An effective PI team will likely have staff filling the following roles:

- **System leader.** This should be someone with the authority to make changes and who can see the larger implications of those changes.
- **Day-to-day leader.** This should be an individual who is active in the PI process every day or on a regular basis.
- **Technical experts.** These should be people who know how systems operate from the inside and can devise concrete solutions.
- **Executive sponsor or systems leader.** This is someone in a management position who can provide resources and remove obstacles (probably someone in the middle management or executive level, as described above).
- **Data analysts.** These are people who know how to filter and analyze data and present them in meaningful ways.

Skill Mix

As you work with people on performance improvement, you'll find that the best suited are those with one or both of these general kinds of skills:

- **Adaptive.** These include leadership skills and the willingness to change the culture of the organization.
- **Technical.** These include skills in generating solutions, putting interventions into action, and interpreting and evaluating the results.

Team Huddles

Many PI teams find the use of huddles appropriate and helpful. Huddles are frequent, short briefings at a set time and place each day or week. You can use huddles to provide a quick status update, share an observation and get advice, pass on helpful information or important news, make or revise plans, or just answer any outstanding questions. One benefit of huddles is that they let frontline staff who can't get away for longer meetings be full participants in PI projects. They also keep things moving—something you want in any PI effort.

WHY DO I NEED TO KNOW THIS NOW?

You need to know what PI personnel resources are available to you before you can start the work.

WHERE DO I START?

- **Learn more.** Find out about any existing or proposed improvement team, including (1) how many people have a full-time commitment, (2) how many others can be called on to provide specialized knowledge, and (3) who can get you more resources when you need them.
- **Work with staff.** If there are holes in your team, survey staff to find individuals with the skills and knowledge you need.
- **Provide training.** As resources permit, conduct recruitment and training sessions.

TOOL

Required Performance Improvement Documents and Data Checklist

KEY CONCEPT

IMPROVEMENT OPPORTUNITIES

It's critical to analyze collected data and translate them into information. The information is used to draw conclusions about performance, to report out to leaders and to staff, to identify improvement opportunities, and to set priorities for those improvement opportunities.

PI Data Reporting

Typically, PI data are collected once and then used for multiple reporting outlets—both internal and external. These data may be reported live in meetings or shared in written reports. Efficient and timely data collection and reporting are important so that everyone is getting the information they need with a minimum of extra effort. (*See* Chapter 8 for information on data reporting.)

Prioritizing Initiatives

Executive-level leaders may refer to data to fulfill their duty of prioritizing PI initiatives. But they might need a little help. The PI team may need to educate those leaders about PI data and processes before asking them which areas to tackle first. Factors to share and consider when prioritizing include the following:

- **Experts.** What are the suggestions from people who deal with performance gaps? These people include the following:
  - Senior leader for quality and safety
  - Patient safety officer
  - Medical director or CMO
  - Clinical leaders
  - Staff nurses and other frontline staff
- **Themes.** Do any of these or other common themes appear in the data?
  - Communication
  - Equipment and supplies
  - Identification (for example, mislabeled specimens)
  - Adverse events (including near misses)
- **Reporting requirements.** Mandatory versus elective— what's involved?
- **Performance gap history.** Are previous or ongoing improvement efforts achieving their goals?

WHY DO I NEED TO KNOW THIS NOW?

You can't get started on improvements until you have a plan to identify PI opportunities and address them. Setting priorities is part of Joint Commission Performance Improvement (PI) standards, as well as the Leadership (LD) standards.

WHERE DO I START?

- **Review documents.** As a new accreditation manager, ask to review any PI plans. Look for the following:
  - All required data collection and reporting processes
  - Relevant analyses and action plans
  - Time frames for each plan to reflect priorities
- **Facilitate processes.** If your organization doesn't already have a standardized method for prioritizing, make that a priority. Some organizations use a coding system.
- **Work with leaders.** Show leaders that you want to—and need to—know about PI opportunities.
  - Review *Sentinel Event Alerts* for potential applicability to your organization. Share the information with the PI team and leaders. Then together identify which recommendations (if any) from the *Sentinel Event Alert* you should consider for implementation.
  - Review your data with leaders and work to reach conclusions about what next steps are indicated by what you identified.
  - Suggest using WalkRounds™ or other similar approaches to encourage leaders to get out on the front line and engage with staff about potential PI project opportunities.

KEY CONCEPT

IMPROVEMENT RECOGNITION

Congratulations! The team's hard work has created real change. The performance at your organization has never been higher. Don't keep the good news to yourself. Remember: Success breeds success.

Acknowledging and Recognizing

There are many ways to heighten awareness of the team's achievement:

- **Share success stories.** Publish an article in your organization's newsletter or create a poster that celebrates the accomplishment. Announce your success on your organization's intranet and on bulletin boards.
- **Give awards.** Present a certificate to an individual or a group that contributed to the project. For example, you might recognize someone who identified a potential safety hazard.
- **Conduct campaigns.** Turning a project into a campaign is particularly effective for organizationwide efforts. Use advertising and marketing strategies and energetic leaders to make the project a high-profile priority.
- **Spread the news.** Submit your story for publication or presentation at a conference.

WHY DO I NEED TO KNOW THIS NOW?

Thanking your team members and publicly recognizing their success is a great motivator. If you determine now how you're going to promote achievements, you can share that with your team to encourage positivity and productivity going forward.

WHERE DO I START?

- **Collaborate with experts.** Enlist public relations professionals at your organization or, if possible, outside agencies to spread the word about successful PI efforts. Use your organization's newsletter as a tool too.

CRITICAL CHALLENGES

Every year The Joint Commission publishes a list of standards that surveyors scored most often in the previous year. The list is broken down for each type of accreditation program, but many of these standards highlight issues that are challenging for all organizations. A review of the trends in these data shows standards that might be challenging as you address performance improvement in your organization.

LACK OF THE "RIGHT" DATA

Data collection and analysis requirements are sometimes more challenging for some types of settings than others. The following standards are frequently found noncompliant in small organizations, such as home care agencies:

- PI.01.01.01: The organization collects data to monitor its performance.
- PI.03.01.01: The organization compiles and analyzes data.

What's the problem? Too much or not enough of the following create the challenges:

- **Too many troubles.** Some programs have such a variety of high-risk or troublesome processes it can be difficult to choose which to focus on first. Many organizations are so overwhelmed by these choices that they don't collect any data or choose to collect data that won't lead to meaningful improvements for their organization.
- **Not enough resources.** Compiling and analyzing data may seem a daunting task for an organization that doesn't have resources to do so.
- **Too many variables.** Data collection and analysis requirements differ between settings and services provided. For example, the data collection standard for home care has many different requirements based on types of home care services the agency provides. Organizations must be careful to use the segment-specific elements of performance (EPs) to guide their choices for data collection (for example, hospice or orthotics and prosthetics) and the setting itself (for example, care recipient residence or facility based); this information is clearly identified in the standards on E-dition.

WHY DO I NEED TO KNOW THIS NOW?

Data collection and analysis are the foundation of PI in any segment of health care. The key is to identify and collect meaningful data that can have a positive influence on your organization's performance. You can't start doing this "sometime soon." It must be now, and it must be ongoing.

WHERE DO I START?

- **Know what data you need.** Identifying the available internal and external data sources and reporting requirements that apply to your organization will help guide much of your data collection activities.
- **Collaborate with experts.** If you can't rely on the data at first, then prioritize opportunities by using PI experts in your organization (or a PI consultant) as well as gap history, common themes, and other factors. At least that will help you determine where to start to collect reliable and meaningful data.

TOOL

Performance Improvement Data Sources Checklist

Test Your Knowledge

1. Which of the following statements are true? (Select all that apply.)
   - ☐ a. Six Sigma is an improvement methodology.
   - ☐ b. Your organization is required to use Plan-Do-Check-Act.
   - ☐ c. Toyota Production System is not an improvement methodology.
   - ☐ d. Your organization may use different improvement methodologies.
2. An organization has had a dozen incident reports associated with mislabeled or unlabeled specimens submitted to the lab. No serious adverse events have occurred, although there have been delays in treatment and diagnosis. What should the next step be?
   - ☐ a. Continue collecting incident reports.
   - ☐ b. Conduct a proactive risk assessment.
   - ☐ c. Conduct a root cause analysis.
   - ☐ d. Do nothing until there is an adverse event.
3. An organization is planning on opening a new clinic to address a patient population with significant access issues. What should the next step be?
   - ☐ a. Collect additional data to make sure access is the only problem.
   - ☐ b. Conduct a proactive risk assessment.
   - ☐ c. Conduct a root cause analysis.
   - ☐ d. Do nothing, since this patient population is migratory.
4. The group that sets the priorities and resources for an organization is/are typically the ___.
   - ☐ a. governing body
   - ☐ b. executive leaders
   - ☐ c. frontline managers
   - ☐ d. staff

(continued)

5. Which of the following is often considered the most challenging part of the improvement process?
   - ☐ a. Getting the group together
   - ☐ b. Finding and fixing the problem
   - ☐ c. Sustaining the improvement
   - ☐ d. Getting resources to do the work
6. Internal benchmarking is when an organization ___.
   - ☐ a. compares data collected with other similar entities
   - ☐ b. compares data collected over time
   - ☐ c. compares data collected over time and with other similar entities
7. Which of the following criteria would be best applied for determining a health care quality improvement initiative? (Select all that apply.)
   - ☐ a. Something that occurs infrequently or never
   - ☐ b. Something that is problem prone
   - ☐ c. Something that is high risk
   - ☐ d. Something that has financial ramifications
8. Ideally, one of the members of an improvement team does the work being assessed or has significant knowledge about how the work is done.
   - ☐ a. True
   - ☐ b. False
9. Leadership rounding is an excellent way to identify improvement opportunities in an organization.
   - ☐ a. True
   - ☐ b. False

Records and Information Technology

CHAPTER 17

THE BIG IDEA

Whether written or electronic, the record of care must provide a complete and accurate account of an individual's care. That care may be compromised if information is missing or errors are present in the record. Keeping health information in the record private and secure is another important consideration during the use and storage of the record.

KEY CONCEPTS

- All About the Record of Care
- Health Information Security
- Verbal Orders
- Informed Consent

THE MANUAL

Following are the relevant Joint Commission E-dition® or *Comprehensive Accreditation Manual* chapters:

- "Information Management" (IM)
- "Record of Care, Treatment, and Services" (RC) [not laboratory]
- "Rights and Responsibilities of the Individual" (RI) [not laboratory]

KEY CONCEPT

ALL ABOUT THE RECORD OF CARE

The Joint Commission requires organizations to keep a complete and accurate record of care for every care recipient. It doesn't matter whether your records are on paper or as part of an electronic health record (EHR) system.

Required Elements

Your organization determines the elements of a complete record of care, but at a minimum it must include demographic and clinical information that allows caregivers to do the following:

- Identify the care recipient
- Support the care recipient's diagnosis and condition
- Justify and document the individual's care, treatment, and services
- Promote continuity of the individual's care among providers

Summary lists. For hospitals, critical access hospitals, and ambulatory care centers, the record of care also may include updated summary lists for care recipients who need continuing ambulatory care services (although summary lists are no longer required). The lists can include any significant medical diagnoses and conditions, operative and invasive procedures, and adverse or allergic drug reactions, as well as current medications, over-the-counter medications, and herbal preparations.

Authentication and Timeliness

Dating, timing, and authentication of record of care entries can be problematic. Surveyors will look for this—not because it's easy to spot but because it's so important to have up-to-date and accurate records.

Unique authentication. Only authorized persons can add entries into the record. And each person must authenticate each entry. Authentication of the record of care can include written signatures and initials. But whether electronic or written, the authentication must be unique to the person, and signatures must be dated and timed.

Thirty-day limit on timeliness. Your organization's policies should specify when an individual's record of care must be completed. But it can't exceed 30 days after discharge (or end of an episode of care). In general, it's best to get the record done as soon as possible to avoid late entries.

Making corrections. No one can alter existing documentation. If corrections are needed, your organization should have an approved, legal process for annotations.

For deemed status. For hospitals and critical access hospitals, information on a care recipient's history and physical exam, with updates, must be in the

Top Challenging Record of Care Standards

The following Medication Management standards and elements of performance (EPs) are those that have recently been frequently cited by Joint Commission surveyors for non-compliance.

Standard	Element of Performance (EP)	Applicable Accreditation Program(s)
RC.02.01.01: The medical record contains information that reflects the patient's care, treatment, and services.	**EP 2:** The medical record contains the following clinical information: • The reason(s) for admission for care, treatment, and services • The patient's initial diagnosis, diagnostic impression(s), or condition(s) • Any findings of assessments and reassessments • Any allergies to food • Any allergies to medications • Any conclusions or impressions drawn from the patient's medical history and physical examination • Any diagnoses or conditions established during the patient's course of care, treatment, and services (including complications and hospital-acquired infections). **For psychiatric distinct part units in critical access hospitals:** The diagnosis includes intercurrent diseases (diseases that occur during the course of another disease; for example, a patient with AIDS may develop an intercurrent bout of pneumonia) and the psychiatric diagnoses. • Any consultation reports • Any observations relevant to care, treatment, and services • The patient's response to care, treatment, and services • Any emergency care, treatment, and services provided to the patient before their arrival • Any progress notes • All orders • Any medications ordered or prescribed • Any medications administered, including the strength, dose, route, date, and time of administration • Any access site for medication, administration devices used, and rate of administration • Any adverse drug reactions • Treatment goals, plan of care, and revisions to the plan of care • Results of diagnostic and therapeutic tests and procedures • Any medications dispensed or prescribed on discharge • Discharge diagnosis • Discharge plan and discharge planning evaluation	Critical Access Hospital

Standard	EP	Applicable Accreditation Program(s)
RC.02.01.01: The patient record contains information that reflects the patient's care, treatment, or services.	**EP 2:** The patient record contains the following clinical information: • Any medications administered, including dose • Any activity restrictions • Any changes in the patient's condition • Any summaries of the patient's care, treatment, or services furnished to the patient's physician or allowed practitioner • The patient's medical history • Any allergies to medications • Any adverse drug reactions • The patient's functional status • Any diet information or any dietary restrictions • Diagnostic and therapeutic tests, procedures, and treatments, and their results • Any specific notes on care, treatment, or services • The patient's response to care, treatment, or services • Any assessments relevant to care, treatment, or services • Physician or allowed practitioner orders • Any information required by organization policy, in accordance with law and regulation • A list of medications, including dose, strength, frequency, route, date and time of administration for prescription and nonprescription medications, herbal products, and home remedies that relate to the patient's care, treatment, or services • The plan(s) of care **For DMEPOS suppliers serving Medicare beneficiaries:** The DMEPOS prescription, any certificates of medical necessity (CMN), and pertinent documentation from the beneficiary's prescribing physician or allowed practitioner.	Home Care

health record within 24 hours after registering or being admitted and before any surgery or procedures using anesthesia.

Accuracy

It's particularly important to make sure the record of care is right whenever an individual visits a health care organization. This can be particularly critical the first time a person visits for care, treatment, or services. Why? Because the information in the record of care is what will be shared whenever individuals make transitions from one provider or setting to another.

WHY DO I NEED TO KNOW THIS NOW?

The records of care for the population(s) you serve are important documents. Knowing how well your organization complies with standards related to them should be one of your priorities. Addressing compliance problems should be a continuous process.

PICTURE THIS

Record of Care

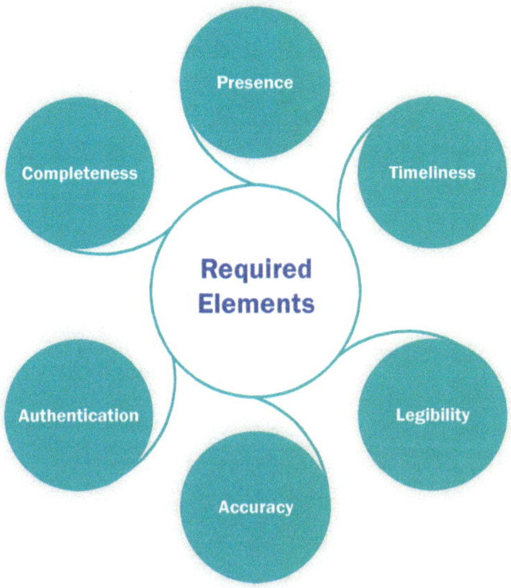

WHERE DO I START?

- **Review documents.** Read your policy to see what it contains about correcting errors in the record of care. If it isn't clear, collaborate with your risk managers or legal counsel about how to annotate errors clearly and legally and ensure that the policy is updated.
- **Check documentation.** Work with your record of care audit team to check documentation of what the team is finding, including authentication and timeliness issues. Work with the performance improvement team to improve your compliance regarding records of care, as needed.
- **Encourage technology use.** Use of EHRs can make data in records even more useful and meaningful—as well as more legible. If your system is set up to allow individuals to download their own records, that's a good start. Incorporating physician dashboards and fostering access via mobile devices is also a progressive route some organizations are using.

TOOL

Point-of-Care Health Records Checklist

PICTURE THIS

Prohibited Abbreviations

Abbreviations, Acronyms, and Symbols	Intended Meaning	Common Misinterpretation
Abbreviations		
AD or AS or AU/ OD or OS or OU	right ear, left ear, each ear right eye, left eye, each eye	mistaken for the opposite abbreviation
cc	cubic centimeters	mistaken as "u" (units)
HS	half strength	mistaken as bedtime
hs	at bedtime, hours of sleep	mistaken as half strength
IJ	injection	mistaken as "IV" or "intrajugular"
IU*	international unit	mistaken as "IV" (intravenous) or 10 (ten)
OD or o.d.	once daily	mistaken as "right eye"
OJ	orange juice	mistaken as OD or OS
Q.D. or QD or q.d. or qd*	every day	mistaken as "q.i.d." (four times daily)
Q.O.D. or QOD or q.o.d. or qod*	every other day	mistaken as "q.d." (daily) or "q.i.d." (four times daily)
q1d	daily	mistaken as "q.i.d." (four times daily)
SC or SQ or sub q	subcutaneous	SC mistaken as "SL" (sublingual) SQ mistaken as "5 every" "q and sub q mistaken as "every"
ss	sliding scale	mistaken as "55"
U or u*	unit	mistaken as the number "0" or "4" or mistaken as "cc"
μg	microgram	mistaken as "mg"
Dose Designations		
"Naked" decimal point (.5 mg)*	0.5 mg	mistaken as "5 mg"
Trailing zero after decimal point (1.0 mg)*	1 mg	mistaken as "10 mg"
Adding a period to an abbreviation (mg. or mL.)	mg or mL	period is unnecessary and may be mistaken as a number if poorly written
Numerical dose and unit of measure run together (10mg or 100mL)	10 mg or 100 mL	"m" is sometime mistaken as a zero
Large dose without comma (100000 units or 1000000 units)	100,000 units or 1,000,000 units	larger numerals are easily mistaken if properly placed comma is missing

(continued)

Abbreviations, Acronyms, and Symbols	Intended Meaning	Common Misinterpretation
Drug Name Abbreviations		
APAP	acetaminophen	not recognized as acetaminophen
CPZ	Compazine (prochlorperazine)	mistaken as chlorpromazine
HTC	hydrocortisone	mistaken as hydrochlorothiazide
$MgSO_4$*	magnesium sulfate	mistaken as morphine sulfate
MS or MSO_4*	morphine sulfate	mistaken as magnesium sulfate
NoAC	novel or new oral anticoagulant	mistaken as no anticoagulant
ZnSO4	zinc sulfate	mistaken as morphine sulfate
Symbols		
x3d	for three days	mistaken as "3 doses"
< or >	less than and more than	mistaken as the opposite intention; incorrect symbol used
Ø or ø or ϕ	zero or null sign	mistaken as "4," "6," "8," and "9"
@	at	mistaken as "2"
&	and	mistaken as "2"
+	plus or and	mistaken as "4"
°	hour	mistaken as "0"

* These abbreviations, symbols, and acronyms are listed in Joint Commission Standard IM.02.02.01, EP 3.

Joint Commission surveyors are still finding orders, preprinted forms, and medication-related documentation with abbreviations, acronyms, symbols, and dose designations that are prohibited in accordance with the list in Standard IM.02.02.01. Included in that list is QD (every day), QOD (every other day), and U (unit). How might the abbreviations and symbols as they are displayed be confusing if they appeared in the health record? The above table identifies what was the intended meaning and what it is misinterpreted as, and recommended corrections.

KEY CONCEPT

HEALTH INFORMATION SECURITY

Keeping health information secure in a time of electronic information goes beyond locking doors and drawers. The US Department of Health and Human Services reports that 707 data breaches occurred in 2022, exposing more than 51.9 million patient records. The most common locations for breaches are network servers and e-mail, with the majority involving hacking or other information technology (IT) incidents. The Joint Commission and state and federal law requires maintaining the privacy and integrity of health information, which may include more than the records of care. Security protocols should address protecting records from loss, theft, damage, destruction, and unauthorized use.

TOOLS

Cybersecurity Risk Assessment Checklist

Health Information Policy Evaluation Checklist

Health Information Policy and Protocols

The Joint Commission requires health care organizations to have a written policy that addresses the security of health information, including access, use, and disclosure. The protocols your organization puts in place in relation to this policy should consider access to the information, sensitivity of the information, and specific exposure risks.

Restricting Access to Health Information

Limiting who can access records of care is part of any information security protocol. Some facilities are open 24 hours; some are not. Some facilities use mainly electronic records; some use a mix of paper-based and electronic information. Regardless, all records should always be locked or monitored, with access limited to authorized individuals—by keys or by passwords.

Health Information Recovery and Continuity

Records are subject to a range of risks. All organizations should have a disaster recovery plan in place to safeguard health information in the event of a disaster or interruption in information processes. Routine backups of electronic records and storage of copies in a secure, separate location are common to most recovery plans. In addition, per the standards, staff should be trained on what to do when information systems are down and how to report a service glitch or gap.

Records Retention

Making sure records retention regulations are followed is another concern. The Joint Commission requires your policies to address retention. But be aware that there may be state regulations for record retention that you need to follow.

WHY DO I NEED TO KNOW THIS NOW?

A large part of your job involves information: accessing it and sharing it for compliance efforts. Protecting information is just as important, so you need to find out sooner rather than later about that and how it affects your job and your organization.

WHERE DO I START?

- **Learn more.** Your organization may be paper based, electronic only, or a mixture. Find out what type of information is stored in what formats and why. This will help you find information when you need it and help you understand how security requirements will work best within your system. Specifically, find out about collection of health information via uniform data sets, required for standardization within your organization.
- **Review documents.** Read through your organization's required policies and related protocols for health information security. Do they seem thorough?
- **Collaborate with experts.** Work with your information management team and facilities services to make sure your organization has a downtime plan for EHRs. Records must always be accessible. This may be part of the utility's management plan and the emergency operations plan/emergency management plan, or it may be a separate plan (see Chapter 10 for additional information on emergency and utilities management plans).

KEY CONCEPT

VERBAL ORDERS

In some cases, a provider is unable to write out medication orders or enter them into an electronic system. The provider instead delivers the orders verbally in person or by telephone, which can cause confusion. Verbal orders may pose a greater risk for miscommunication, misinterpretation, and error.

PICTURE THIS

Health Insurance Portability and Accountability Act (HIPAA) and Protected Health Information (PHI)

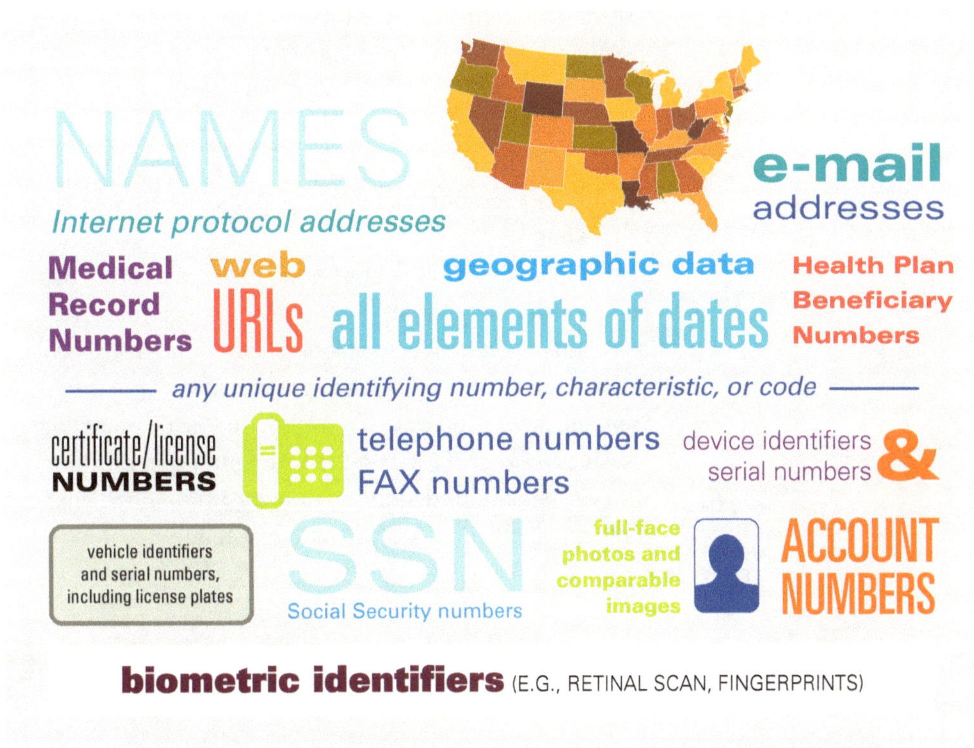

The HIPAA Privacy Rule by the National Institutes of Health is a comprehensive federal protection for the privacy of protected health information (PHI). PHI is a subset of overall health information that might be collected in an organization. Understanding that concept is an important part of health information security. PHI should be secure while still allowing the flow of health information to ensure high-quality care.

PHI that's linked based on the above 18 identifiers must be treated with special care for privacy and security.

De-identifying for data use. Under HIPAA, PHI can be stripped of identifiers (known as de-identifying) to use the data for research and other purposes (such as for performance improvement data). This is done by two methods: (1) the removal of the 18 specific identifiers, *and* (2) having a statistical expert validate and document that the statistical risk of re-identification is very small.

Limiting Verbal Orders

The best way to avoid confusion caused by verbal orders is to limit or eliminate them. If physicians are on site, they should write out or electronically input the orders. When off site, they can input them via remote access to an electronic health information system, if it's set up that way. Some organizations prohibit verbal orders except for emergencies, while others allow them with written follow-up orders within a set time frame. In any case, your organization does have to decide who is permitted to receive and record verbal orders, per law and regulation.

Authentication

All verbal orders must be documented, or authenticated, with dates and names of everyone involved in the order—who ordered it, received it, recorded it, and followed it. And all verbal orders must be authenticated within the time frame allowed by law and regulation and the organization's policy. The documentation/authentication of verbal orders must—in most program settings—include the time the order was received when required by law and regulation (for example, in the case of deemed status organizations).

WHY DO I NEED TO KNOW THIS NOW?

Use of verbal orders is one of those things you can focus on quickly. On-the-spot standards training for easy-to-spot compliance issues is often the best way to deal with some problems, including this one.

WHERE DO I START?

- **Perform audits.** Conduct regular audits on verbal orders; record and share the results.
- **Work with staff.** Survey staff and providers about reasons for failure to comply with verbal order procedures (for example, fatigue or workload, communication challenges, look-alike/sound-alike medications). Share the results and solicit suggestions for addressing the issues, including use of "read-backs." Avoid pointing fingers and focus on finding solutions.
- **Celebrate success.** Recognize when staff and providers consistently comply with verbal order procedures. Bringing attention to such a success may motivate and inspire staff to continue the trend.

KEY CONCEPT

INFORMED CONSENT

Informed consent agreements are a critical component of the health record. But note: Informed consent is not simply a signed agreement in which a care recipient grants permission to have a procedure performed; it's a process. That process is aimed at a mutual understanding of what is involved in the individual's care, treatment, and services. Consideration of care recipient needs and preferences, care recipient education, and involving the care recipient in decisions about their health care are all included in that process.

Organization Policy

The Joint Commission requires all organizations (except laboratories) to have a written policy on informed consent. It needs to include the following:

- Specific procedures that require informed consent (per law and regulation) and any conditions for exceptions to getting informed consent
- A description of the process for obtaining informed consent, including how it's documented in the care recipient's health record
- When surrogate decision-makers can give informed consent

Informed Consent Process

The process itself is required to include a discussion with the care recipient about the proposed care, treatment, and services—including risks, side effects, likelihood of achieving care goals, possible recuperation problems, alternatives, and conditions that might require disclosure or reporting of care recipient information.

Care recipient communication needs. An important part of that discussion is assessing the care recipient's expectations regarding information delivery and decision-making. Specifically, care recipients might need to know the rationale behind informed consent, and they might want to involve others in the decision-making process. Informed consent information should be presented in a way the care recipient understands; ensuring this understanding may prompt the need for interpreting services or translated documents. (*See* "Rights and Responsibilities of Care Recipients" in Chapter 9 for more information.)

Signed and dated. The care recipient's understanding is authenticated with their signature, including the date and time. Adding the time shows the signature is secured before the procedure requiring informed consent is initiated.

WHY DO I NEED TO KNOW THIS NOW?

Informed consent issues (including legal ones) can be minimized if you take the initiative to help make the process clear to staff and the individuals you serve. It's something surveyors will look for because obtaining informed consent properly is important for ensuring the safety and rights of the individuals you serve.

WHERE DO I START?

- **Check documentation.** Look at some informed consent forms and see how the process is documented—and by whom. Perform audits of your own informed consent documents and consider the following during the process:
  - Is the dating and timing of signatures in line with your policies?
  - Have the potential risks and benefits of the procedure been discussed?
  - Were the care recipient's communication needs and preferences met?
  - Are translated documents provided for care recipients who have a preferred language other than English? Was an interpreter used to help the care recipient ask questions?
  - Are witnesses involved?
  - Can the forms be improved?

"I heard that...

informed consent for invasive procedures is only applicable to the inpatient setting."

fact:

Informed consent is required beyond the inpatient setting. For example, invasive procedures performed at an ambulatory surgery center require it. Invasive procedures performed at an office-based surgery practice also require informed consent if the practice's own policy requires it.

- **Collaborate with experts.** Work with patient rights advocacy groups or your legal department to develop a structured program to guide staff, providers, and care recipients through the informed consent process. Make sure it addresses care recipients with language barriers, varying literacy needs, and technology barriers (such as use of an online form). Also check state laws and regulations, as they vary state to state.

"I heard that...

electronic health records prevent all medical errors."

fact:

EHRs do not prevent all medical errors. Although machines often make processes more efficient, people may still input incorrect or incomplete information, forget to input it, or fail to input it in a timely manner. Glitches in technology can also lead to errors. An incomplete interface of electronic systems across departments or between organizations, power outages, and system backup failures can all lead to lost information. However, electronic records systems have many benefits. For example, instant access to important and complete care recipient information can help providers better diagnose and treat illnesses more immediately and effectively. Other benefits include the ability to interface with various departments and organizations, access to computerized provider order entry (CPOE) systems, monitoring of safety issues, and organization of administrative clinical data and demographics.

CRITICAL CHALLENGES

Every year The Joint Commission publishes a list of standards that surveyors scored most often in the previous year. The list is broken down for each type of accreditation program, but many of these standards highlight issues that are challenging for all organizations. A review of the trends in these data shows one standard that might be challenging as you audit records of care in your organization.

COMPLETE AND ACCURATE HEALTH RECORDS

Who's tackled this compliance challenge successfully? Many health care organizations find this a challenge, but home care organizations (12%) struggle to maintain compliance with Record of Care, Treatment, and Services (RC) Standard RC.02.01.01.

What's the problem? These main factors contribute to health record noncompliance tagged by surveyors:

- **Lack of clarity in records.** Although staff can often articulate the reason why particular aspects of care, treatment, or services are being provided to a care recipient, that isn't always clear in the health record. The required element of justification is often missing, perhaps because it seems obvious to caregivers.
- **Lack of information in records.** Sometimes there's not enough information documented in the health record to support the care recipient's diagnosis and to justify the care provided. It is important to collect detailed information and to make it available to all those involved in providing care.
- **Human error.** Plain old mistakes are a big contributing factor. Staff may forget that all entries in the health record need to be dated, for example.

WHY DO I NEED TO KNOW THIS NOW?

What if your health records were perfect? It's a lofty but attainable goal. If you can visualize it now and get leaders to support that vision, you can pursue this critical and highly visible issue and make at least some progress toward perfection.

WHERE DO I START?

- **Encourage technology use.** If possible, encourage the use of electronic records in your organization. This technology can help flag missing information in your health records, particularly demographic information. It can also help ensure that all portions of the record are in one place and easily accessible to staff. Use of a failure mode and effects analysis (FMEA) to support the transition is recommended (see "Performance Improvement Approaches" in Chapter 16).
- **For measurement submissions.** The submission format for delivering some types of data to The Joint Commission—including the US Centers for Medicare & Medicaid Services (CMS), OASIS (Outcome and Assessment Information Set) data for home care, Minimum Data Set (MDS) data for nursing care centers, and meaningful use data for Accountable Care Organizations (ACOs)—and other regulators must be electronic.

Test Your Knowledge

1. During a mock survey observation, a physician asks a nurse to give a mumps, measles, and rubella (MMR) vaccine to a patient. The nurse prepares and administers the MMR vaccine. The nurse documents what was given in the medical record. Which of the following is a correct statement?
   - ☐ a. The provider telling the nurse to administer the MMR vaccine is a verbal order.
   - ☐ b. No order is required because the patient was due to receive this vaccine.
   - ☐ c. If the provider documents this in the progress notes, no order is required.
2. The Joint Commission requires health care organizations to use electronic records.
   - ☐ a. True
   - ☐ b. False
3. Which of the following statements is correct?
   - ☐ a. Medications prescribed by outside providers do not need to be added to the medical record.
   - ☐ b. An organization can develop its own Do Not Use abbreviation list, separate from The Joint Commission's list.
   - ☐ c. Informed consent refers to the process and the form.
   - ☐ d. If you cannot produce requested documentation during a survey, you cannot be cited for this on a survey.
4. During a care recipient tracer, care recipient labels were found in the regular trash. Staff explained that the labels were found when they were cleaning out the tray table drawer after the care recipient was discharged two days ago. Which of the following statements is correct regarding privacy and information security?
   - ☐ a. There is not an issue because the care recipient is no longer under the care of the organization.
   - ☐ b. This is a HIPAA privacy and information security issue.
   - ☐ c. This would be an issue if the labels got into the wrong hands.
   - ☐ d. There is not an issue because the labels had the care recipient's name, date of birth, and medical record number.
5. Which of the following could be an information privacy issue? (Select all that apply.)
   - ☐ a. The pharmacy staff announces care recipient and medication names when ready for pickup.
   - ☐ b. A computer screen in a clinic hallway is active.
   - ☐ c. A care recipient's medication administration record printout is left on a breakroom table.
   - ☐ d. A staff member is talking in detail about the care recipients they are in charge of while standing in line at a coffee kiosk.
6. Which of the following could govern how long medical records are retained by an organization? (Select all that apply.)
   - ☐ a. Care recipient preference
   - ☐ b. Provider preference
   - ☐ c. Federal and state regulations
   - ☐ d. Organization policies and procedures

Staffing

CHAPTER 18

THE BIG IDEA

The quality and safety of the care, treatment, and services delivered by a health care organization depends directly on its staff and licensed practitioners. Because of this, the orientation, training, and competency assessment of those staff and licensed practitioners are critical. So are the recruitment of providers and the processes used to determine their qualifications and competencies—as well as what practices they're permitted to perform in your health care organization.

KEY CONCEPTS

- Sufficient and Well-Trained Staff
- Staff Qualifications and Competencies
- Credentialing and Privileging/Permitting Practitioners
- Nursing Services

THE MANUAL

Following are the relevant Joint Commission E-dition® or *Comprehensive Accreditation Manual* chapters:

- "Human Resources" (HR) [not behavioral health care and human services]
- "Human Resources Management" (HRM) [behavioral health care and human services only]
- "Leadership" (LD)
- "Medical Staff" (MS) [critical access hospitals and hospitals only]
- "Nursing" (NR) [critical access hospitals and hospitals only]

PRIORITY

WorkforceSafety and Well-Being

COVID-19 exacerbated the global shortage of health care workers and the challenges they face—including accelerated rates of mental health crises. As shortages of health care workers continue, creating strain on these professionals, quality and safety risks often rise. The Joint Commission is working to address contributing factors of strain such as overly burdensome administrative requirements. In that spirit, we are reviewing all of our "above and beyond" requirements, those that go beyond the US Centers for Medicare & Medicaid Services (CMS) Conditions of Participation (CoPs) and are not on crosswalks to the CoPs.

The ultimate outcome is to eliminate standards and elements of performance (EPs) that don't add commensurate value and in doing so supporting our workforce, which is one of our top ongoing priorities.

TOOL

Required Staff Education and Training Checklist

KEY CONCEPT

SUFFICIENT AND WELL-TRAINED STAFF

In recent years health care organizations have faced severe staff shortages and difficulties keeping sufficient and well-trained staff. In fact, it's created a threat to care recipient safety and quality in many cases.

The Right Number and Type of Staff

You can't just stretch your staff or replace them with other, less-qualified employees. Without sufficient staff, care recipient flow can slow to a crawl. Staff caseloads can become unmanageable. Without qualified staff, lives are endangered. Having the right number and the right type of staff on duty improves care recipient safety and care quality.

Developing staffing plans. The standards require your organization to have the administrators, supervisors, and staff necessary to support its services. That takes planning as well as the flexibility to adjust plans when services or staffing needs change. Nursing management and other leaders are in charge of developing staffing plans.

Orientation, Training, and Education Requirements

Having the right number and the right type of staff still isn't enough. You also need to make sure they're doing the right things in the right ways. Even the most qualified staff need orientation and supervision, as well as ongoing education and training.

Orientation and education topics. Although requirements may differ for each health care setting, the following are common orientation and education topics:

- **Orientation topics**
  - Key safety content (orientation before staff provide care, treatment, or services)
  - Policies and procedures related to job duties and responsibilities
  - Specific job duties and responsibilities
  - Sensitivity to cultural diversity based on job duties and responsibilities
- **Education topics**
  - Skills and knowledge to maintain or increase competency
  - Skills and knowledge whenever changes in responsibilities require education specific to care recipient needs
  - Rights of the care recipient, including the ethical aspects of care, treatment, and services

The standards and elements of performance (EPs) on E-dition are sorted by accreditation program setting. You can use the search function to search for any standards or EPs that include training or education requirements by using the search terms *train*, *orient*, *assess*, and *educate*.

Top Challenging Staffing Standards

These staffing standards and elements of performance (EPs) are those that have recently been most frequently cited by Joint Commission surveyors as non-compliant.

Standard	Element of Performance (EP)	Applicable Accreditation Program(s)
HR.01.06.01: Staff are competent to perform their responsibilities.	**EP 18:** The staff member's competency assessment includes the following: • Direct observations of routine patient test performance, including patient preparation, if applicable, and specimen collection, handling, processing, and testing • Monitoring, recording, and reporting of test results • Review of intermediate test results or worksheets, quality control, proficiency testing, and preventive maintenance performance • Direct observation of performance of instrument maintenance function checks and calibration • Test performance as defined by laboratory policy (for example, testing previously analyzed specimens, internal blind testing samples, external proficiency, or testing samples) • Problem-solving skills as appropriate to the job	Laboratory
HR.01.06.01: Staff are competent to perform their responsibilities.	**EP 20:** After the first year of employment, each staff member's competence is assessed on an annual basis for all laboratory tests they perform. This assessment is documented.	Laboratory
HR.02.01.04: The organization permits licensed practitioners to provide care, treatment, and services.	**EP 1:** Before permitting licensed practitioners new to the organization to provide care, treatment, and services, the organization does the following: • Documents current licensure and any disciplinary actions against the license available through the primary source. • Verifies the identity of the individual by viewing a valid state or federal government–issued picture identification (for example, a driver's license or passport). • Obtains and documents information from the National Practitioner Data Bank (NPDB). The medical director evaluates this information. • Determines and documents that the practitioner is currently privileged at a Joint Commission–accredited organization; this determination is verified through the accredited organization. If the organization cannot verify that the practitioner is currently privileged at a Joint Commission–accredited organization, the medical director oversees the monitoring of the practitioner's performance and reviews the results of the monitoring. This monitoring continues until it is determined that the practitioner is able to provide the care, treatment, and services that they are being permitted to provide.	Nursing Care Center
HRM.01.02.01: The organization verifies and evaluates staff qualifications.	**EP 1:** The organization performs primary source verification of staff licensure, certification, or registration in accordance with law and regulation and organization policy at the time of hire and the time of renewal.	Behavioral Health Care and Human Services
HRM.01.06.01: Staff are competent to perform their job duties and responsibilities.	**EP 3:** The organization conducts an initial assessment of staff competence. This assessment is documented.	Behavioral Health Care and Human Services

WHY DO I NEED TO KNOW THIS NOW?

If your organization is understaffed and/or has staff that are poorly oriented and trained, it's going to affect everything you do. It will negatively affect your organization's ability to provide safe, high-quality, and effective care to those you serve. It's also going to compromise compliance with Joint Commission accreditation.

WHERE DO I START?

- **Conduct tracers.** Find out if you have problems with care recipient flow, work flow, or other functions affected by staffing levels by incorporating questions about sufficient staffing into your mock tracers.
- **Collaborate with experts.** If necessary, work with senior managers, your performance improvement team, and human resources (HR) personnel to examine the relationship between clinical functions and processes and staffing at your organization. Is more training needed? A different staffing mix?
- **Check documentation.** Make sure staff education requirements are being met by reviewing personnel files with your HR department.

KEY CONCEPT

STAFF QUALIFICATIONS AND COMPETENCIES

Care recipients need to trust that all staff are qualified and competent. You need to be able to trust that's the case too—for compliance reasons and more. For that assurance, you must be able to rely on HR staff and those in charge of training employees.

HR Tracking Processes

HR staff are responsible for tracking the qualifications and competencies of most staff. Licensed practitioners are tracked by a medical staff office in hospitals and critical access hospitals, whereas they are tracked by HR in other accreditation programs (*see also* "Credentialing and Privileging/Permitting Practitioners" in this chapter). This involves a variety of processes, including the following:

- **Verifying qualifications.** This is done for nearly all staff. Typically, primary source verification (or verification from a designated equivalent source) is used when required. For licensed practitioners, a primary source verification is required. For nonlicensed practitioners, a reliable secondary source is acceptable.
- **Assessing competency.** Competency requires three attributes: knowledge, technical skills, and ability. Assessments are conducted at orientation and at regular periods, per the standards, for all staff to validate that they can competently apply the knowledge and technical skills to perform required tasks.
- **Monitoring contracted services.** Standards for this are in the "Leadership" chapter, but internal management or HR may monitor the work of these employees (*see* Chapter 14 for additional information relating to leadership responsibilities).

WHY DO I NEED TO KNOW THIS NOW?

Knowing what HR does regarding staff qualifications and competencies will give you insight into staff skills. That can be helpful in so many ways, including knowing how to find out which staff might be best able to help with compliance issues—or who might be well qualified to serve on an accreditation committee (see Chapter 3 for additional information about accreditation committees).

WHERE DO I START?

- **Review documents.** Sit down with HR staff to review their processes and the types of documents they use for tracking qualifications and competencies. Ask questions. Listen. Share the Joint Commission requirements to make sure no records are lacking or incomplete. Then suggest working together to correct any issues, including scheduling of regular records reviews.

KEY CONCEPT

CREDENTIALING AND PRIVILEGING/PERMITTING PRACTITIONERS

Every organization needs to have a process for confirming the qualifications and competencies of individuals permitted by law and the organization to practice independently. In hospital settings, this process of verifying qualifications and defining responsibilities is known as credentialing and privileging and is handled by the medical staff office. In many nonhospital settings, the process for verifying qualifications and competencies for these individuals is performed by designated staff members and is addressed by HR staff. In nursing care centers, for example, this responsibility may be delegated to the administrator or a committee of the governing body.

Clinical Privileges

Clinical privileges for licensed practitioners are granted by a governing body, such as a board, in certain settings.

For nonhospital settings: In ambulatory care and office-based surgery settings, leaders grant privileges.

For hospital settings: In hospitals and critical access hospitals, privileges are based on recommendations from the organized medical staff. Other providers, such as physician assistants (PAs) and advanced practice registered nurses (APRNs) also are credentialed and privileged through the medical staff process if they are providing a medical level of care and decision-making.

Competency Reviews

After granting privileges or permitting practitioners to provide care, treatment, and services, your organization needs to perform regular competency reviews of providers—in accordance with the standards, applicable laws, and your own

COMPETENCY VS. EDUCATION AND TRAINING

Training, education, and competency are aspects of the process of making sure you have qualified staff. Though they may sound similar, they are not synonymous.

- **Education.** The process of receiving systematic instruction resulting in the acquisition of theoretical knowledge.
- **Training.** The process of gaining specific—often manually performed—technical skills.
- **Competency.** A combination of observable and measurable knowledge, skills, abilities, and personal attributes that constitute an employee's performance. Competency differs from education and training in that competency incorporates all three attributes—knowledge, technical skills, and ability—and all are required to deliver safe care and correctly perform technical tasks.

Assessing competency, then, is the process by which the organization validates, via a defined process, that an individual can perform a task, consistent with the education and training provided.

Orientation is a term paired with *competency* in the standards that also can be misunderstood. Orientation is defined by The Joint Commission as "a process used to provide initial training and information while assessing the competence of clinical staff relative to job responsibilities and the organization's mission and goals."

It may further be described as an introductory program and/or set of activities intended to guide a person as they adjust to new surroundings, employment, policies/procedures, and so on. Each organization is responsible for determining when and how long an individual is considered to be in "orientation."

policies. These reviews are used to determine whether any clinical privileges or allowable practices need to be revised and if they should be renewed. Staff with the educational background, experience, or knowledge related to the skills being reviewed assess competence. Organizations should establish the review variables: how often they're conducted, what kind of practice data are collected, how the data are used, who reviews them, who makes decisions based on them, and so on.

OPPE and FPPE. In hospitals and critical access hospitals, two types of formal practice evaluations are required for medical staff: ongoing professional practice evaluation (OPPE) and focused professional practice evaluation (FPPE). OPPE is continual (as defined by your organization) and addresses performance of clinical privileges for all providers privileged through the medical staff processes. FPPE is done to assess a specific practice by a specific individual when that individual is granted new privileges or a performance issue is identified or triggered.

The FPPE process must be predefined and consistently implemented for all newly requested privileges. Both qualitative and quantitative data should be considered when designing the process.

Qualitative data might include information from periodic chart reviews, types of care recipient complaints, peer recommendations, descriptions of procedures performed, and so on. They are data collected primarily through discussion and observation and are often non-numerical.

Quantitative data, on the other hand, are numerical data that may include measures such as length of stay trends, postprocedure infection rates, rate of compliance with core measures, and so on.

Medical Staff Bylaws

In hospitals and critical access hospitals, all medical staff at your organization (including licensed practitioners with clinical privileges) are subject to the organization's medical staff bylaws. The organized medical staff uses the bylaws to define how the medical staff functions.

WHY DO I NEED TO KNOW THIS NOW?

You need to ensure that staff working in your health care organization are properly qualified. To accomplish this task, you need to be aware of the policies and procedures for credentialing and privileging, or the permitting of licensed practitioners to provide care, in your organization.

WHERE DO I START?

- **Review documents.** If you're working in a hospital or critical access hospital, evaluate the medical staff bylaws as well as the credentialing and privileging processes to make sure that they meet Joint Commission Medical Staff (MS) requirements. In other health care settings, compare your process for assessing the competency of licensed practitioners to provide care, treatment, and services to the requirements set forth in the "Human

Resources" (HR) or "Human Resources Management" (HRM) chapter on E-dition or in your *Comprehensive Accreditation Manual*.

- **Facilitate processes.** If your organization doesn't have a clear performance monitoring review process for medical staff or licensed practitioners, sit down and help staff work it out. You'll learn more about the process and build relationships with medical staff. Critical questions to ask: Do any privileged providers meet the glossary definition of *staff* as found on E-dition or in your *Comprehensive Accreditation Manual*? If privileged providers are direct or contract employees, do the HR policies apply to them or does the HR policy default to the medical staff processes (in hospitals and critical access hospitals)?
- **Check documentation.** Make sure all credentialing and privileging processes are properly documented. If a provider's credentials are called into question, can a recent review of that person's qualifications and performance be provided? If privileges based on changes need to be expedited, is there a process in place for that? These are questions you need to ask HR and the medical staff office (if appropriate) to ensure compliance and care recipient safety and quality.

"I heard that...

The Joint Commission mandates a particular number of charts or data elements for FPPE and OPPE."

fact:

According to Standards MS.08.01.01 and MS.08.01.03 for hospitals and critical access hospitals, your organization and organized medical staff decide which indicators and what methodology to use. For example, they choose whether to use direct observation, chart audits, communication with other staff, or information technology data, as well as the number of activities to evaluate and what should be tracked within the categories. It all depends on what needs to be assessed for each individual.

KEY CONCEPT

NURSING SERVICES

Solid nurse leadership + qualified nursing staff = excellent care of the individual. Nurse leaders and executives must stay on top of the latest research and evidence-based practices and incorporate them into the policies and procedures of the nursing staff. That's just one reason why so many organizations value these nurse leaders.

Responsibilities and Skills

Nurse executives in hospitals are responsible for overseeing the nursing budget, productivity, care recipient safety and satisfaction, staff retention, and nursing policies and procedures. Clinical nurse managers in other settings may provide oversight for staff assignments, coordinate care and referrals, and ensure that care recipient needs are continually assessed and that individualized plans of care are developed, implemented, and updated. Clearly, today's nurse leader, or nurse executive, must have expertise in a variety of areas, including the following:

- Strategic planning
- Negotiating
- Budgeting
- Marketing
- Trend variance analysis
- Information technology

TOOL

Credentials Verification Record

Nurse Staffing

In nonhospital settings, where there may not be a nurse leader or nurse executive, the organization must plan nurse staffing (RN, LPN, CNA) based on the following applicable elements:

- Acuity of the care population(s)
- Complexity of clinical tasks
- Staff experience and expertise
- Physical layout of the facility or number of visited sites
- Personal care needs of the care recipients
- Varying cognitive levels of the population(s) served
- Level of supervision needed to maintain care recipient safety

WHY DO I NEED TO KNOW THIS NOW?

Nurses are primary partners in accreditation. The sooner you get to know your nurses, the sooner you can begin to nurture relationships that will help nursing services meet standards critical to high-quality care—and to maintaining compliance.

WHERE DO I START?

- **Collaborate with experts.** Nurse leaders and nurse executives are experts in so many areas. Find out more about how you can collaborate with them on compliance issues. Start by finding out whether the leadership structure of your organization gives nurse leaders or nurse executives primary control when it comes to nursing activities.
- **Attend and observe.** Job shadow a nurse leader or nurse executive for even one day and you'll see how vital they are to your organization. Then take time to job shadow other nurses to develop relationships supportive of your accreditation efforts.

CRITICAL CHALLENGES

Every year The Joint Commission publishes a list of standards that surveyors scored most often in the previous year. The list is broken down for each type of accreditation program, but many of these standards highlight issues that are challenging for all organizations. A review of the trends in these data shows three standards that might be challenging as you address staffing in your organization.

VERIFYING QUALIFICATIONS

Verifying staff qualifications as required by Human Resources Management (HRM) Standard HRM.01.02.01 continues to be a challenge for behavioral health care and human services (6%).

What's the problem? Confusion arises due to the following:

- **Licensed versus nonlicensed staff.** Primary source verification is required for licensed employees. But for nonlicensed staff, verification doesn't have to come from a primary source.
- **Requirements from multiple states.** Different states have different requirements for licensure, criminal background checks, and health care screenings. So things can get complicated if your organization has locations in multiple states.

WHY DO I NEED TO KNOW THIS NOW?

Surveyors aren't going to accept an excuse that verifying qualifications is confusing. You need to help your organization figure out how to make any confusing processes less confusing.

WHERE DO I START?

- **Facilitate processes.** Find out if HR uses qualification verification checklists for positions in your organization. These types of helpful checklists could include details on specific primary sources required as well as checks for individual state requirements. HR should include which primary sources may be used to verify specific types of licenses and other qualifications.

MEASURING COMPETENCY

Measuring staff competency, as required by Human Resources (HR) Standard HR.01.06.01 (HRM.01.06.01 in behavioral health care and human services), is a particular challenge for the behavioral health care and human services, home care, and laboratory settings.

What's the problem? Assessment is difficult for different reasons in these settings:

- **More than a license.** For behavioral health care and human services providers, it's all about the regular and ongoing interactions with specific individuals they serve. Just checking a license isn't enough. Supervisors need to observe how their staff communicate with the people they care for. Also, competencies may differ by population. For instance, is the staff person trained to work with children? Does the person know how to assess suicide risk? Is the person competent in safe and appropriate use of restraint or seclusion?
- **Limited experts.** In a home care program, there may be only one staff person in each area of expertise—one social worker, one physical therapist, and so on. The challenge is in finding another person familiar with and competent in that area to assess competencies.
- **Off-site assessment.** In laboratories, the biggest challenge may be that a lot of nonwaived testing (that is, moderate and high-complexity

testing) is done outside the lab by nonlab personnel. For instance, respiratory therapists might test blood gases. But everyone performing those tests, even if they aren't lab staff, must have their lab competencies assessed. (*See* Chapter 19 for more on waived testing.)

WHY DO I NEED TO KNOW THIS NOW?

Understanding the reasons for challenges in measuring competency at other organizations can help you focus on what can be done to solve similar problems in your organization.

WHERE DO I START?

- **Collaborate with experts.** HR and the medical staff office are the experts on competencies and performance evaluation. But you need to make sure requirements are met. For example, in lab settings, are recommendations from the US Food and Drug Administration, Clinical Laboratory Improvement Amendments of 1988, and/or the US Centers for Medicare & Medicaid Services being used as required for competencies? Are competencies objective and quantifiable? Are forms complete enough? Sit down with HR and the medical staff office to discuss any problems they're having meeting Joint Commission requirements.
- **Conduct tracers.** If competency assessment comes up on tracers, consult with your performance improvement team to see about getting projects to address these issues. Staff competency is not something to set aside for later.
- **Network with peers.** If you're in a setting with limited staff in an area of expertise, check with your peers at other organizations. Perhaps an arrangement can be made to use that expert.

GRANTING PRIVILEGES

Compliance with Standard HR.02.01.03 is required for ambulatory care and office-based surgery, and Standard HR.02.01.04 is required for nursing care centers. These standards address granting clinical privileges to licensed practitioners (ambulatory care and office-based surgery) and permitting licensed practitioners to provide care, treatment, and services (nursing care centers). It's been a challenge for organizations in those settings for several years. In some years, it's been the top challenging standard.

What's the problem? It's different for different settings, as follows:

- **Objective measures.** As noted in the challenges for competency standards, the work is nearly all interaction with care recipients. That can make it more difficult to objectively determine if a person's performance meets the requirements of their clinical privileges.
- **Too few or too transient staff.** Many larger health care organizations have multiperson departments to oversee all the checks required to

meet this requirement. Nursing care centers and other smaller facilities may not. Also, nursing care centers tend to hire a lot of entry-level employees and have a high rate of turnover, so it can simply be hard to keep up.

WHY DO I NEED TO KNOW THIS NOW?

When your organization grants someone clinical privileges or permits them to practice, it's essentially saying, "We trust you to treat our care recipients." It's part of your job to make sure that's really the case.

WHERE DO I START?

- **Encourage technology use.** Software can be invaluable in situations in which forms are overwhelming and staff numbers are underwhelming. Be supportive of any staff efforts to get new technology to help them.
- **Review documents.** Check to see that your organization has developed solid processes and objective measures for determining competency in areas where quality of interaction is assessed. For example, determine the following:
  - Do chart reviews indicate that the provider is providing accurate diagnoses?
  - Does the provider use the SMART (**S**pecific, **M**easurable, **A**chievable, **R**easonable, and **T**ime-bound) treatment planning approach?
  - Does the provider use reflective listening?
  - Does the provider note other risk factors?
  - Does the process involve an objective provider to make such judgments?
  - Does a formalized list of "triggers" exist that would require a provider to be monitored and/or have privileges reconsidered?
- **Check documentation.** Make sure all staff and licensed practitioners are credentialed, privileged, qualified, and competent, per Joint Commission standards, by reviewing your documentation against the requirements.

Test Your Knowledge

1. According to Joint Commission requirements, how frequently must performance evaluations be conducted?
   - ☐ a. Semiannually
   - ☐ b. Annually
   - ☐ c. Biennially
   - ☐ d. Triennially
2. Performance evaluation and competency assessment are the same.
   - ☐ a. True
   - ☐ b. False
3. During the review of credentialing, staff stated that a licensed practitioner presented a letter from their licensing board. Staff accepted this as proof of current licensure and no additional steps were needed. Which of the following statements are correct?
   - ☐ a. This describes primary source verification.
   - ☐ b. To be valid, the letter needs to be notarized.
   - ☐ c. This is not primary source verification.
   - ☐ d. The department chair still needs to vouch for the practitioner.
4. Primary source verification can be conducted by which of the following means? (Select all that apply.)
   - ☐ a. A letter from the agency
   - ☐ b. An e-mail from the agency
   - ☐ c. A phone call with the agency
   - ☐ d. Use of an authorized agency website
5. In hospitals and critical access hospitals, the document(s) that governs how the organized medical staff interacts with the hospital is called ___. (Select all that apply.)
   - ☐ a. medical staff bylaws
   - ☐ b. governing body bylaws
   - ☐ c. rules and regulations
   - ☐ d. chief of staff memorandums
6. During a care recipient tracer, a medical assistant's point-of-care testing (POCT) competency assessment was done by the clinic manager. The clinic manager has an MBA and an MPH. The clinic manager has not been certified for POCT. What should the organization do? (Select all that apply.)
   - ☐ a. Have a medical assistant from another clinic perform the competency assessment.
   - ☐ b. Get a staff member with POCT competency to conduct the assessment.
   - ☐ c. Nothing else is needed as long as the clinic manager can document the competency assessment.

(continued)

(continued)

7. Which of the following describes a focused professional practice evaluation (FPPE)?
   - ☐ a. It is a Joint Commission hospital and critical access hospital requirement.
   - ☐ b. It is applied continuously while a medical staff member is practicing at a hospital.
   - ☐ c. It looks at a practitioner's entire practice at an organization.
   - ☐ d. It is a process that reviews a practitioner's practice prior to working at the current organization.

Testing and Transplants

CHAPTER 19

THE BIG IDEA

Laboratory tests are commonly used to provide information about a care recipient's health. A laboratory's quality system and proper documentation of these procedures are critical to ensure accuracy of lab results. The same kind of attention to detail is part of the processes involved in organ and tissue transplants—documentation and tracking of care recipient and donor information are essential.

KEY CONCEPTS

- Waived Testing
- Quality Control Checks
- Transplants

THE MANUAL

Following are the relevant Joint Commission E-dition® or *Comprehensive Accreditation Manual* chapters:

- "Quality System Assessment for Nonwaived Testing" (QSA) [laboratory only]
- "Transplant Safety" (TS) [not applicable to assisted living community, behavioral health care and human services, home care, or nursing care centers]
- "Waived Testing" (WT)

Top Challenging Waived Testing Standards

These waived testing standards and elements of performance (EPs) have been recently cited frequently by Joint Commission surveyors as non-compliant.

Standard	Element of Performance (EP)	Applicable Accreditation Program(s)
WT.03.01.01: Staff and licensed practitioners performing waived tests are competent.	**EP 5:** Competency for waived testing is assessed using at least two of the following methods per person per test: • Performance of a test on a blind specimen • Periodic observation of routine work by the supervisor or qualified designee • Monitoring of each user's quality control performance\ • Use of a written test specific to the test assessed	Nursing Care Center
WT.04.01.01: The organization performs quality control checks for waived testing on each procedure.	**EP 4:** For instrument-based waived testing, quality control checks are performed on each instrument used for patient or resident testing per manufacturers' instructions.	Nursing Care Center

KEY CONCEPT

WAIVED TESTING

The Clinical Laboratory Improvement Amendments of 1988 (CLIA '88) define three levels of complexity among laboratory tests, from high complexity to waived testing, the most common type of point-of-care testing (POCT) performed by health professionals. Waived tests are easy-to-administer, fairly low-risk tests, such as ovulation, blood glucose, dipstick or tablet reagent urinalyses, and rapid strep tests. The list of methods that are approved as waived is under constant revision, so it is advisable to check the manufacturer's instructions and the US Food and Drug Administration's (FDA) waived test database. A link to that database appears in "Recommended Resources" at the end of this book.

CLIA Certificate of Waiver

Any organization in any setting needs a CLIA Certificate of Waiver before it's allowed to conduct any waived tests. It doesn't matter how few or how many tests you perform, or even whether or not you charge the care recipient.

POCT leader. The CLIA certificate should identify the individual responsible in your organization for policies and procedures related to waived testing, usually a laboratory director. That person also designates in writing who can perform waived tests. If your organization doesn't have a POCT program managed by laboratory medicine, you'll need to consult with laboratory leaders.

Per the manufacturer. Waived tests must be performed in accordance with the manufacturer's instructions, or the test isn't waived and all regulatory requirements for nonwaived tests would then apply. No modifications, shortcuts, or exceptions are allowed.

Performing Waived Testing

Waived tests include test systems cleared by the FDA for home use and those tests approved for waiver under the CLIA criteria. Joint Commission standards apply to staff performing waived testing using instruments belonging to the staff member, the organization, or the care recipient.

Qualification and competencies. For nonwaived testing, the requirements are detailed and specific. Waived testing, on the other hand, has few requirements. Under Joint Commission standards, the individuals performing the tests need to be qualified and competent, and the person who deems them as such must also be qualified and competent. In addition, individuals performing the test must follow all applicable state laws and regulations.

Documentation, Documentation, Documentation

Waived tests must be documented along with quality control (QC) results, including internal and external controls for waived testing. The results are entered into the care recipient's record of care. Though not required, documentation should include the following:

- Two care recipient identifiers
- Date of testing
- Test kit lot number
- Test result
- Testing personnel identifier

WHY DO I NEED TO KNOW THIS NOW?

Even though waived testing is (by definition) simple, accurate, and safe, there's still risk of error or harm to the care recipient. Knowing about risks—even seemingly small ones—and complying with requirements to manage them is what your job is all about.

WHERE DO I START?

- **Check documentation.** Be sure your organization has proper, up-to-date certification to perform the types of testing you do. The US Center for Medicare & Medicaid Services (CMS) site provides a downloadable form and instructions for applying for CLIA certification (see "Recommended Resources" near the end of this book).
- **Work with leaders.** Find out more about who's involved in your POCT program or if you have to help set one up. Use an organizational flowchart to help clarify who is reporting to whom. Then identify the leaders you'll be interfacing with most often.

KEY CONCEPT

QUALITY CONTROL CHECKS

Because there are so many different waived tests and they're performed by so many different staff, QC checks are vital. The Joint Commission requires these checks for instrument-based as well as non–instrument-based waived testing.

"I heard that...

having an MD exempts a provider from waived testing competency requirements."

fact:

The Joint Commission requires everyone who performs even the simplest waived testing to demonstrate at least two methods of competency per person per test, including physicians.

QC Plan and Checks

A QC plan, created by the person named on your organization's CLIA certificate, must include directives for QC checks. The plan should spell out QC needs for each type of test, based on the following:

- How the test is used
- Reagent stability
- Manufacturer's instructions
- Organization's experience with the test
- Currently accepted guidelines

QC Documentation

Like waived testing itself, QC checks on those tests must also be documented; unlike the tests, the checks don't have to be in the record of care. Failure to perform QC testing correctly and according to each manufacturer's instructions—and to document test results reliably and accurately—could contribute to incorrect diagnoses, inappropriate or unnecessary medical treatment, and poor outcomes for care recipients.

WHY DO I NEED TO KNOW THIS NOW?

Understanding the needs and responsibilities for proper QC of waived testing is important because so many caregivers may be performing such tests. You need to be sure every one of them is doing everything correctly, for the sake of safety of the care recipient and your organization's accreditation status.

TOOL

Self-Assessment Checklist for Good Waived Testing Practices

WHERE DO I START?

- **Facilitate processes.** Meet with staff to discuss barriers to QC documentation. Be sure to address documentation of QC results as well as where the documentation is filed and managed (including backup for electronic storage).
- **Provide education.** Staff who perform waived testing may not be as aware of the potential risks as they should be. Working with your POCT leader, create a program to provide frequent up-to-date education on the risks.

KEY CONCEPT

TRANSPLANTS

Organ and tissue transplants can enhance or save lives. If not performed with the utmost care, however, they can cost lives.

Donation, Procurement, and Transplant

For hospitals that offer transplant services, staff may be dealing with recipients, donors, and their families. In addition, the organization may have an agreement with an organ procurement organization (OPO) for procurement of solid organs, eyes, and tissues, or it may choose to use an OPO, along with an eye bank and tissue bank. Policies and procedures and staff education are part of the donation and procurement process too. Sensitivity and discretion are paramount. But so are clear, standardized procedures to help the process run smoothly and safely. Joint Commission standards clearly delineate between the donation or procurement of both organs and tissues (TS.01.01.01) and transplanting organs (TS.02.01.01) or tissues. Standard TS.03.01.01 addresses standardized procedures for overseeing the acquisition, receipt, storage, and issuance of tissues throughout the hospital, while TS.03.02.01 addresses the tracing of tissues. Standard TS.03.03.01 focuses on the investigation of tissue adverse events.

Transplant Infection Risk

Infections contracted through contamination during transport, storage, or handling are all too real. And the number of transplants is increasing, which increases the risk of infection.

WHY DO I NEED TO KNOW THIS NOW?

Much of what you do requires working with a variety of people following somewhat complex rules. Add to this the time-sensitive nature of many transplants. Making sure standardized procedures are followed to reduce risks is something you need to be prepared to champion.

WHERE DO I START?

- **Review documents.** Organizations that store or use tissue must have policies and procedures for identifying, tracking, storing, and handling the tissues—and reporting any tissue adverse events. Look for ways to standardize any procedures.
- **Conduct tracers**. Transplants are a perfect candidate for tracers. Focus on one aspect—such as bidirectional tracking—or on the whole process.
- **Work with leaders.** To make improvements in the organ procurement and transplant process, you may want to work with performance improvement leaders to conduct a failure mode and effects analysis (FMEA) (*see* Chapter 16).

TOOL

Tissue Adverse Events Investigation Procedures

CRITICAL CHALLENGES

Every year The Joint Commission publishes a list of standards that surveyors scored most often in the previous year. The list is broken down for each type of accreditation program, but many of these standards highlight issues that are challenging for all organizations. A review of the trends in these data shows two areas of focus that may be challenging as you address waived testing compliance in your organization.

WAIVED TESTING COMPETENCIES

Nursing care centers and office-based surgery practices struggle to comply with Waived Testing (WT) Standard WT.03.01.01, which requires staff performing waived tests to be competent.

What's the problem? Most times, the problem is not competence, but demonstrating it. Some providers believe that their license or experience exempts them from competency assessments. Also, some organizations use only one of the four approved competency assessment methods, when two are required. Finally, the individuals responsible for providing orientation and training and assessing competency don't always fully understand waived testing.

WHY DO I NEED TO KNOW THIS NOW?

Competency needs to be demonstrated for every practitioner who performs waived testing of any sort. You have to help raise awareness of that on a regular basis. You can start right away by educating yourself on this issue and sharing what's in this chapter.

WHERE DO I START?

- **Work with staff.** Consult with human resources to make sure orientation materials include information about waived testing competencies. Then check with the organized medical staff (for hospital settings) to make sure medical staff understand their responsibilities regarding waived testing. If possible, coordinate with the laboratory director to ensure that waived testing practices are in compliance with CLIA requirements and the organization's policy.
- **Conduct tracers.** Checking waived testing competencies can be done as part of tracers on POCT.

NONWAIVED TESTING

Accuracy in nonwaived testing is the goal of the Quality System Assessment for Nonwaived Testing (QSA) standards for those tests. And as with waived testing, documentation is important: Document and Process Control (DC) standards support the QSA standards. QSA and DC standards are unique to Joint Commission Laboratory Accreditation Program settings. Most requirements are based on the CLIA '88 regulations. The remaining are Joint Commission requirements based on clinical best practices and developed by using an expert consensus process.

QSA REQUIREMENTS

The QSA section forms the heart of the laboratory manual, addressing most of the technical aspects of a clinical laboratory. QSA requirements cover proficiency testing (testing of unknown samples to verify the accuracy and reliability of laboratory tests), general quality testing (on tests, methods, and instruments, including calibration testing), and

PICTURE THIS

Nonwaived and Waived Testing

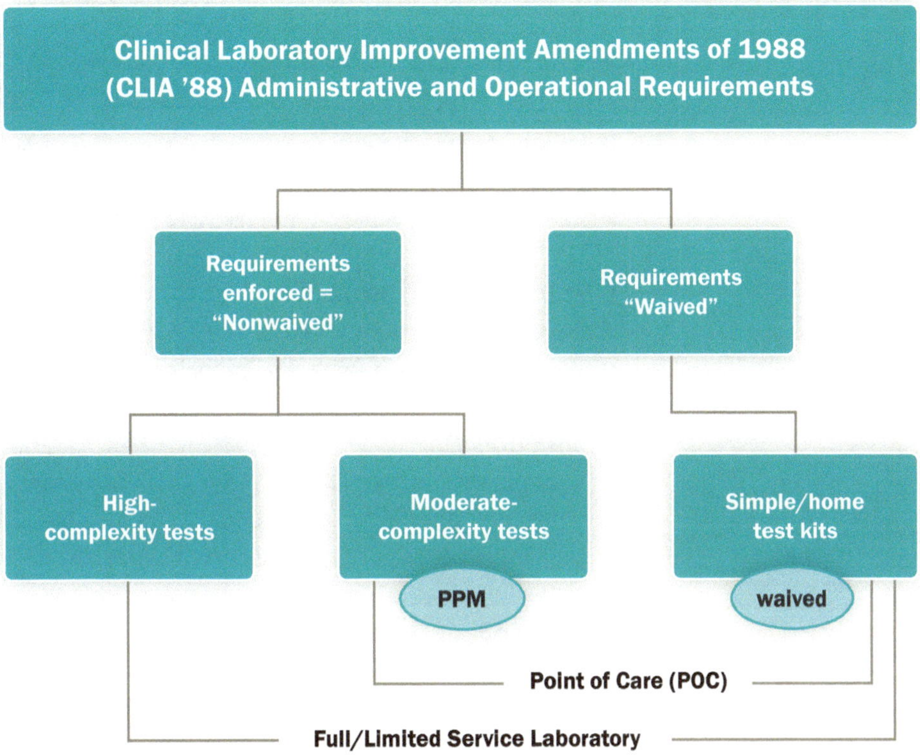

PPM = provider-performed microscopy.

The Clinical Laboratory Improvement Amendments of 1988 (CLIA '88) established regulations that apply to laboratories processing human materials for medical purposes. All laboratories must be either CLIA-exempt or CLIA-registered and certified. And all certified laboratories must comply with CLIA's basic administrative and operational (technical) requirements. CLIA certification covers waived and nonwaived testing (moderate- to high-complexity nonwaived tests, including provider-performed microscopy [PPM] procedures testing, which are covered under the standards in the Laboratory Accreditation Program). The diagram shows which tests can be performed in which circumstances or settings.

specialty and subspecialty testing. Other chapters in the laboratory manual cover other technical requirements of the lab as well, such as the DC chapter.

For deemed status. Laboratories with deemed status must participate in a CMS-approved proficiency testing program that meets regulatory requirements for all specialty and subspecialty testing performed.

NONWAIVED TESTING COMPLIANCE REQUIREMENTS

Due to the technical nature of the requirements for nonwaived testing, you may not be as involved with these standards as with others; you may instead be working with a laboratory director to monitor compliance.

WHY DO I NEED TO KNOW THIS NOW?

If your laboratory is accredited by The Joint Commission, you're responsible for working with laboratory leaders to ensure compliance.

WHERE DO I START?

- **Learn more.** You can find out more about nonwaived testing to work better with your laboratory director. Numerous resources are available to provide detailed technical guidance, such as those available from the Clinical and Laboratory Standards Institute (CLSI) and AABB.
- **Review documents.** Take time to look at your organization's required policies and procedures regarding nonwaived testing, including information within those about required competencies.

Test Your Knowledge

1. According to the Centers for Medicare & Medicaid Services, any clinical site performing laboratory testing must comply with which of the following?
   - ☐ a. American Society of Quality
   - ☐ b. Clinical Laboratory Improvement Amendments of 1988
   - ☐ c. ISO 9000
   - ☐ d. *The Comprehensive Accreditation Manual for Laboratory and Point-of-Care Testing (CAMLAB)*

2. Every ___ performing clinical laboratory tests must have a CLIA registration.
   - ☐ a. practitioner
   - ☐ b. medical assistant
   - ☐ c. location
   - ☐ d. building

3. According to Joint Commission standards, which of the following are required for a point-of-care testing competency assessment? (Select all that apply.)
   - ☐ a. The assessment must be documented at orientation.
   - ☐ b. The assessment must be documented at least annually.
   - ☐ c. The assessment must be conducted by using at least two of the four methodologies.
   - ☐ d. The assessment must be conducted by the clinic's medical director.

4. According to Joint Commission standards, which of the following are required for quality control of waived testing?
   - ☐ a. It must be conducted by a clinical laboratory scientist.
   - ☐ b. It must be completed before each test.
   - ☐ c. It must follow manufacturer's instructions for use.
   - ☐ d. It must be documented in writing.

5. Joint Commission Transplant Safety standards apply only to solid organs that come from humans.
   - ☐ a. True
   - ☐ b. False

6. Which of the following are requirements for a laboratory test to be defined as "waived"?
   - ☐ a. The test needs to be performed by a laboratory scientist.
   - ☐ b. The test requires multiple reagents and sophisticated equipment.
   - ☐ c. The test must be performed at bedside by trained staff.
   - ☐ d. The test takes less than two minutes to perform.

7. Which of the following statements are true?
   - ☐ a. If your organization does not use tissue, the Transplant Safety standards are not applicable.
   - ☐ b. The risk of transplants becoming contaminated during transport, storage, or handling is very low.
   - ☐ c. Staff handling tissue do not require special instructions or competencies.

Recommended Resources

The Joint Commission

2024 Joint Commission Publications

Accreditation and Certification Compliance

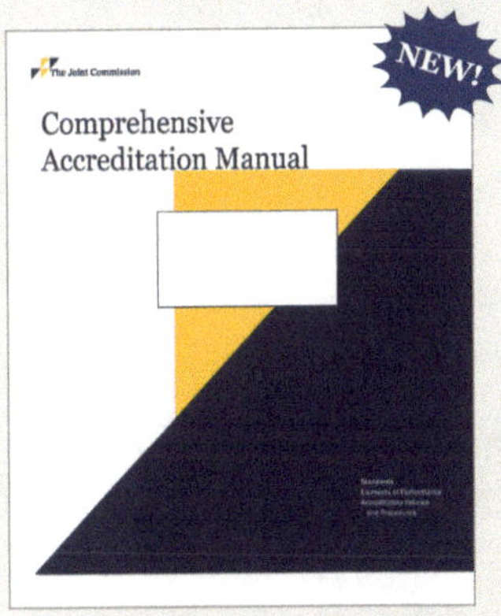

2024 Comprehensive Accreditation Manuals
for Hospital, Ambulatory Care, Assisted Living Community, Behavioral Health Care and Human Services, Critical Access Hospital, Home Care, Laboratory, Nursing Care Center
CAH24, CAC24, EBALC24, CBHC24, CAMCAH24, CAHC24, CLSM24, EBCNCC24
Available as book and/or e-book. Check webstore for your program.

2024 Accreditation Standards Books
for Hospital, Ambulatory Care, and Behavioral Health Care and Human Services
Abridged—includes all standards and other requirements, but no nonscored chapters
HS24, ACS24, BHCS24

2024 Update Services (replacement pages for *CAM* binder) for Hospital, Behavioral Health Care and Human Services
CAH24S, CBHC24S

New Certification Programs!

2024 Health Care Equity Certification Manual
EBHCEC24

2024 Sustainable Healthcare Certification Manual
EBSHCC24

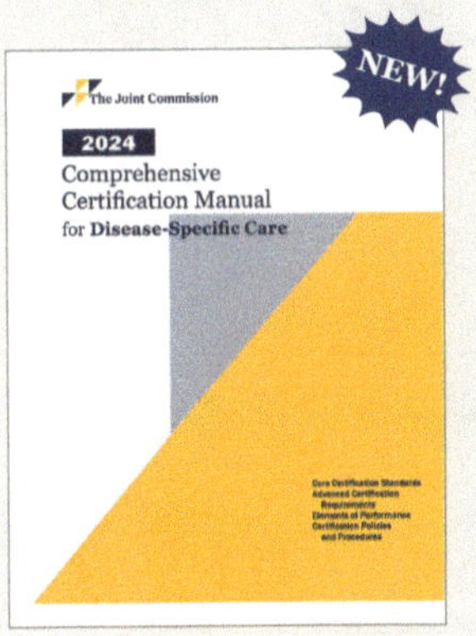

2024 Comprehensive Certification Manual for Disease-Specific Care Including Advanced Programs for DSC Certification
EBDSCC24

2024 Certification Standards Books
for Stroke Certification, Orthopedic Certification
Abridged—includes all standards and other requirements, but no nonscored chapters
SCS24, OCS24

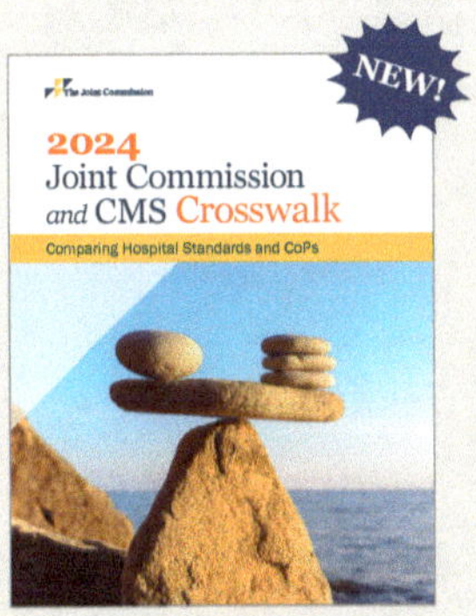

2024 Joint Commission and CMS Crosswalk
CMSX24

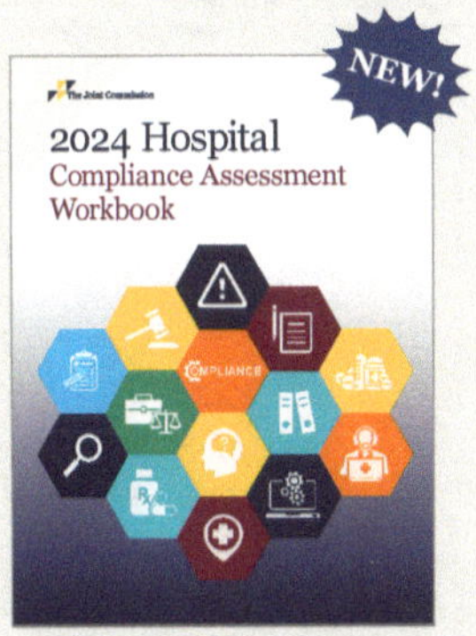

2024 Hospital Compliance Assessment Workbook
HCAW24

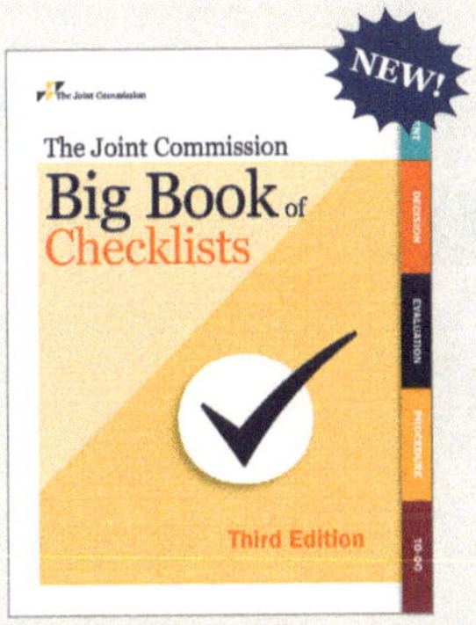

The Joint Commission Big Book of Checklists, Third Edition
JCCHK23

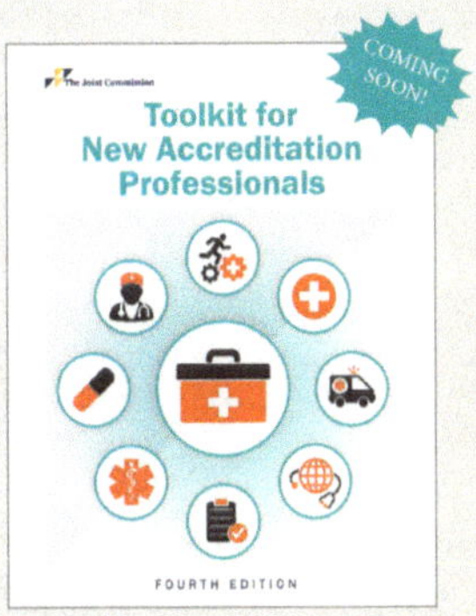

Toolkit for New Accreditation Professionals, Fourth Edition
TNAP24

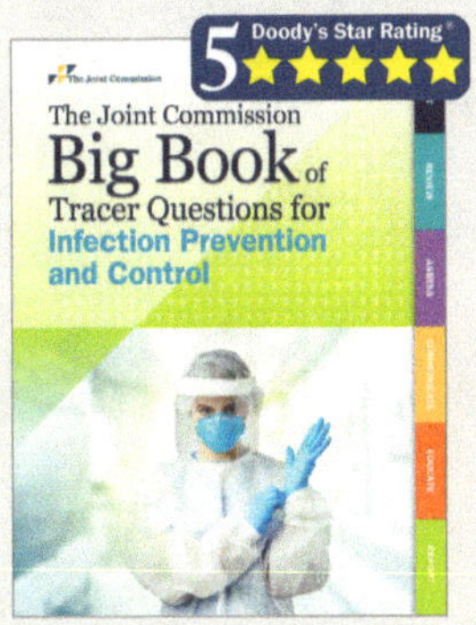

The Joint Commission Big Book of Tracer Questions for Infection Prevention and Control
TQIC21

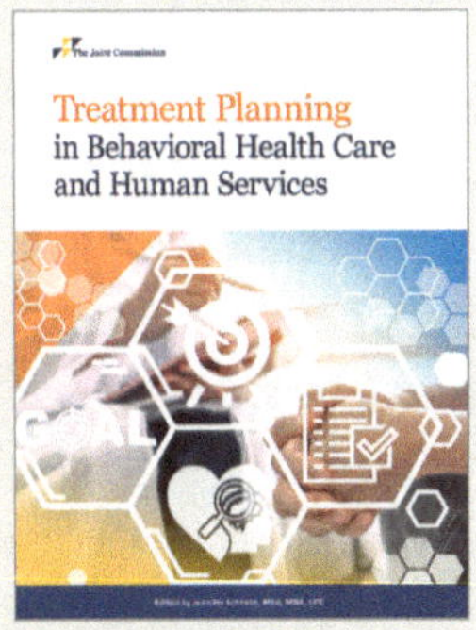

Treatment Planning in Behavioral Health Care and Human Services
TPBH21

PolicySource™: P&Ps for Compliance with Joint Commission Requirements

BEST SELLER!

Policy Source™ 2024

- Hospital/Critical Access Hospital
- Behavioral Health Care and Human Services
- Home Care
- Ambulatory Care/Office-Based Surgery
- Laboratory
- Nursing Care Center/Assisted Living Community

Digital Learning Center

BEST SELLER!

Subscribe to a special collection of JCR's top compliance resources—webinars, videos, newsletters, e-books, and *PolicySource*—all in one place and all at one price, and for your whole team.

DIGITAL LEARNING CENTER

Environment of Care®, Life Safety, and Emergency Management

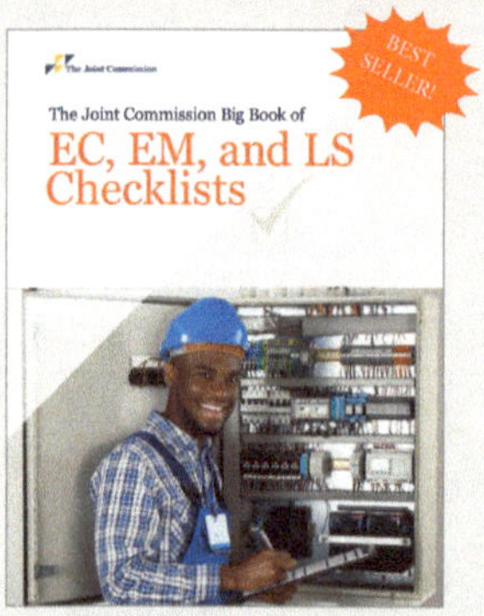

The Joint Commission Big Book of EC, EM, and LS Checklists

JCCHKEC21

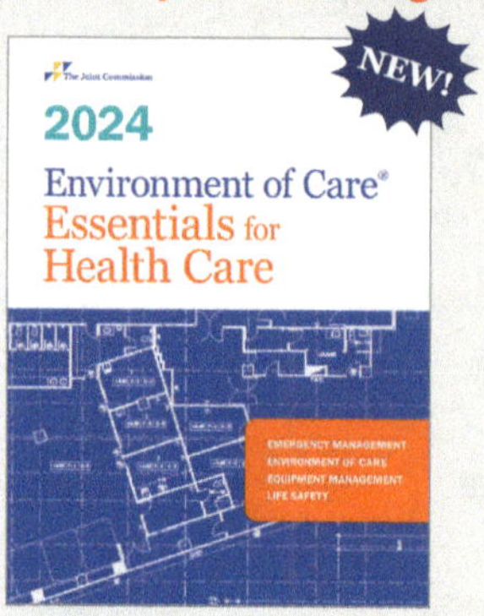

2024 Environment of Care® Essentials for Health Care

ECE24

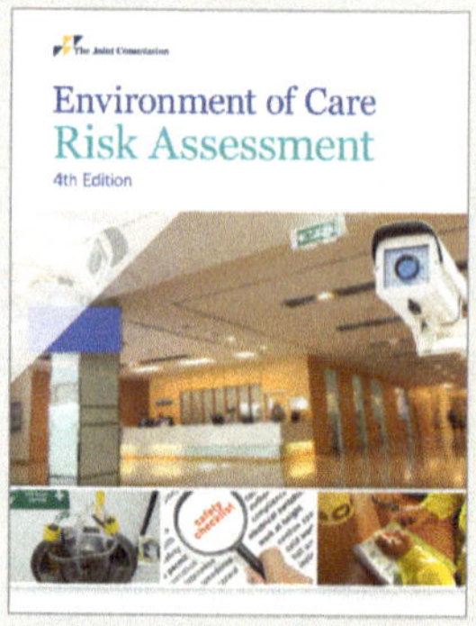

Environment of Care Risk Assessment, Fourth Edition

ECRA22

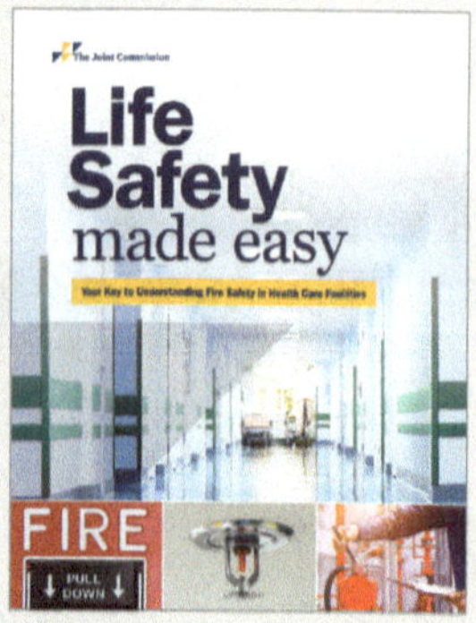

Life Safety Made Easy: Your Key to Understanding Fire Safety in Health Care Facilities

LSME20

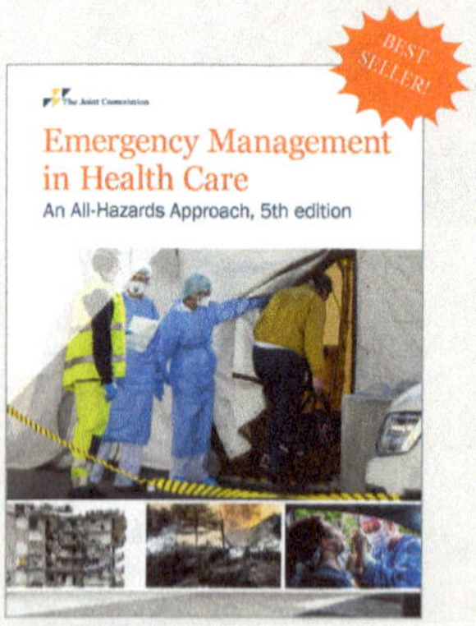

Emergency Management in Health Care: An All-Hazards Approach, Fifth Edition

EM21

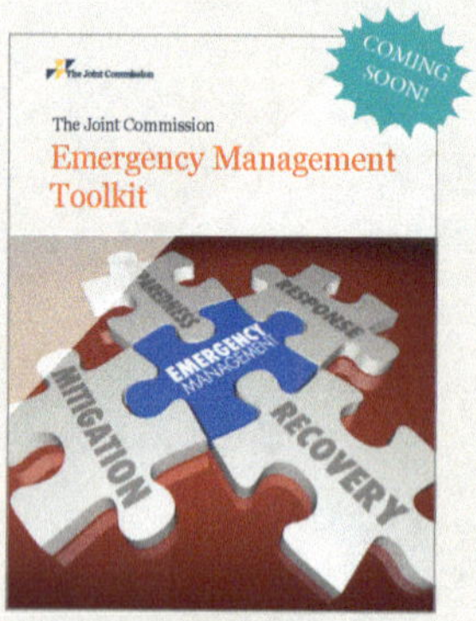

The Joint Commission Emergency Management Toolkit

EMTK24

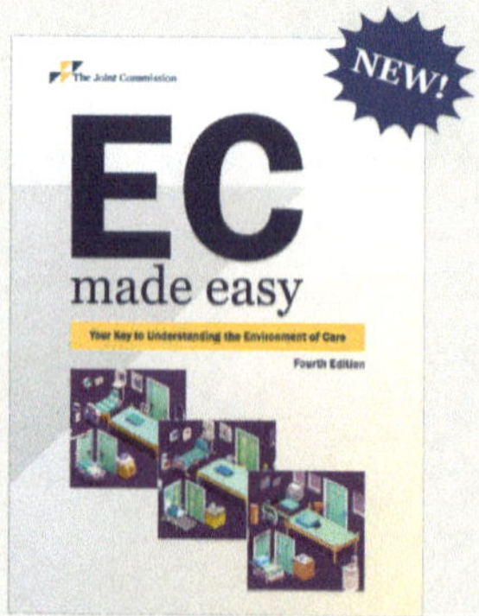

EC Made Easy: Your Key to Understanding EC, EM, and LS, Fourth Edition

ECME23

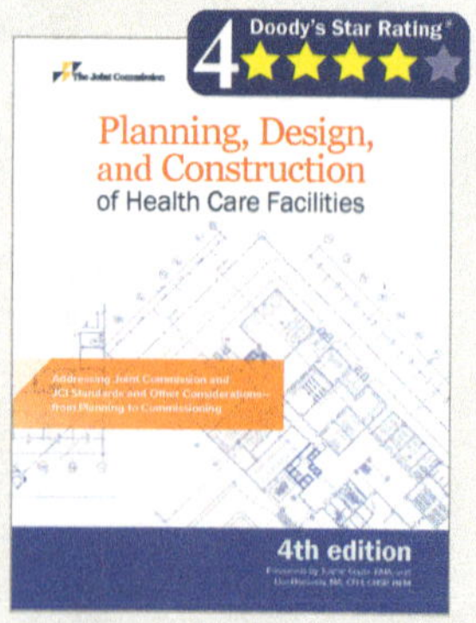

Planning, Design, and Construction of Health Care Facilities, Fourth Edition

PDC19

Infection Prevention and Control

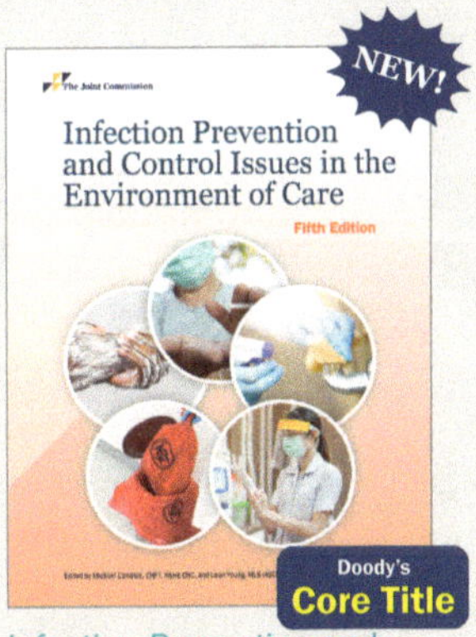

[Infection Prevention and Control Issues in the Environment of Care, Fifth Edition]

IPIEC23

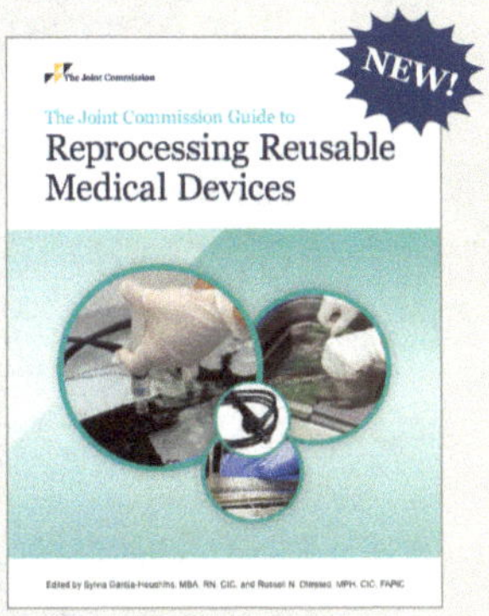

[The Joint Commission Guide to Reprocessing Reusable Medical Devices]

CDS21

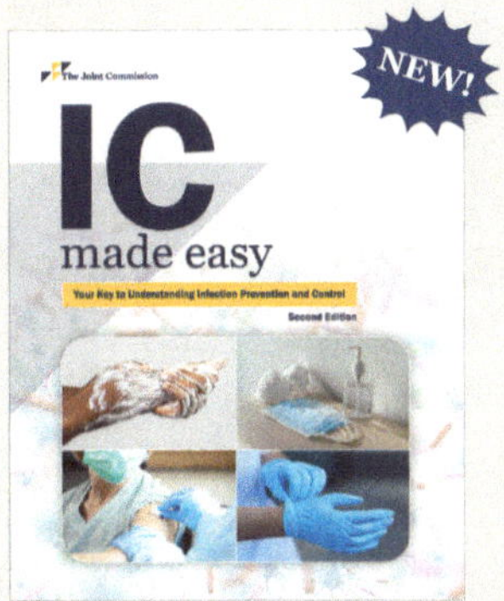

[IC Made Easy: Your Key to Understanding Infection Prevention and Control, Second Edition]

ICME23

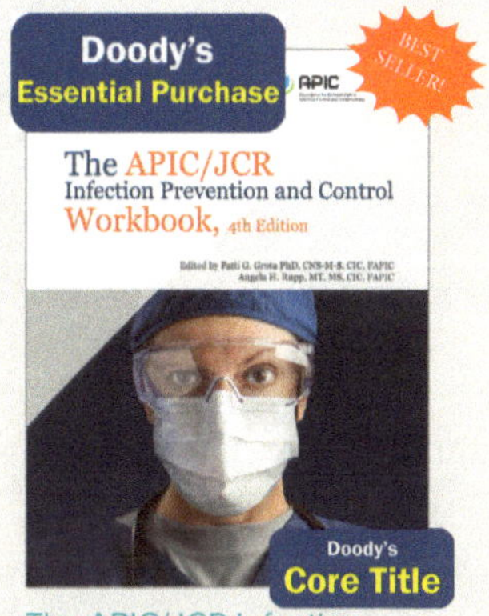

[The APIC/JCR Infection Prevention and Control Workbook, Fourth Edition]

ICSA20

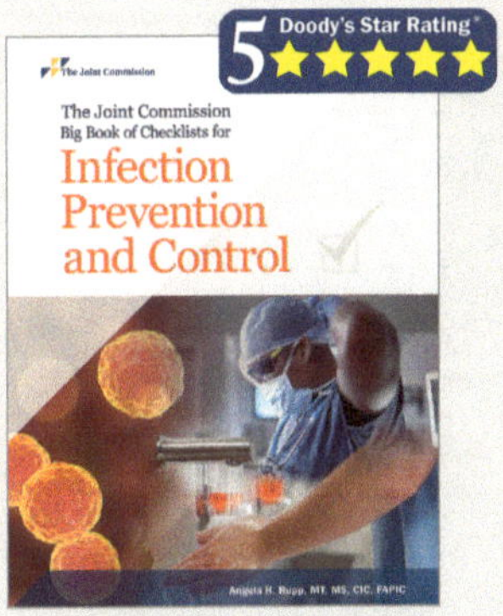

[The Joint Commission Big Book of Checklists for Infection Prevention and Control]

JCCHKIC20

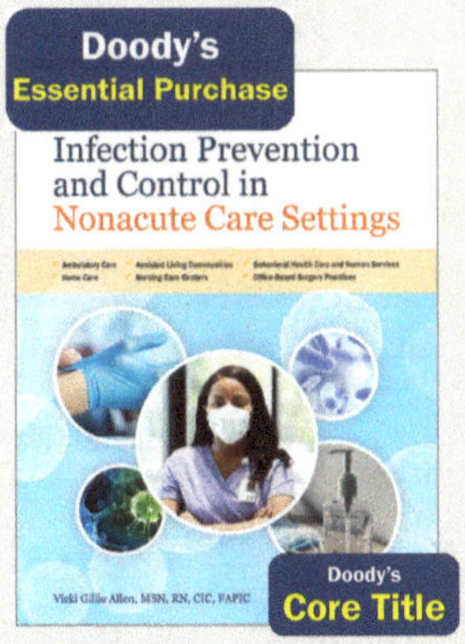

[Infection Prevention and Control in Nonacute Care Settings]

ICNH21

Performance Improvement and Patient Safety

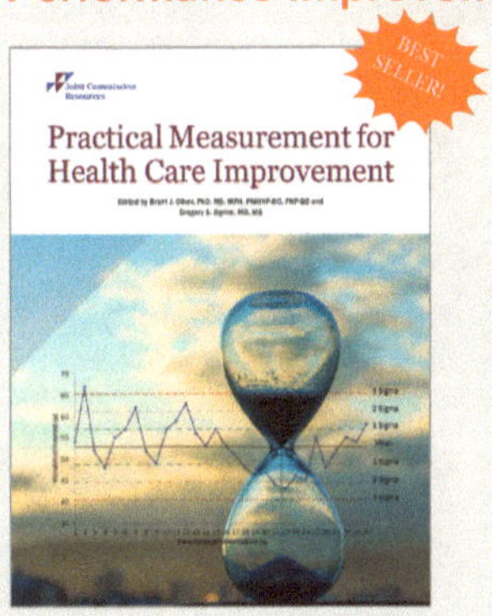

[Practical Measurement for Health Care Improvement]

PPM22

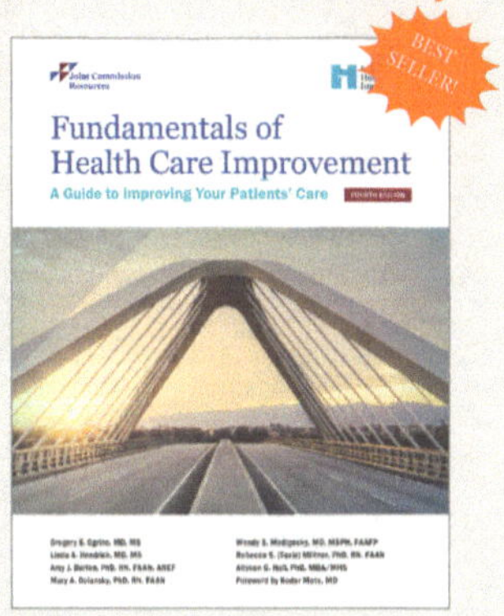

[Fundamentals of Health Care Improvement: A Guide to Improving Your Patients' Care, Fourth Edition]

FHCI22

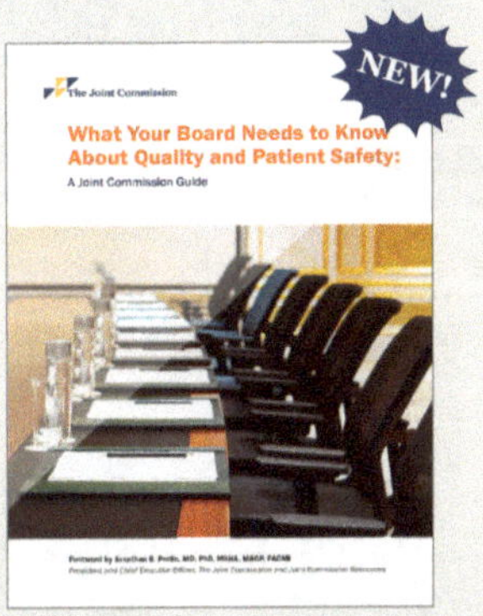

[What Your Board Needs to Know About Quality and Patient Safety: A Joint Commission Guide]

GBB23

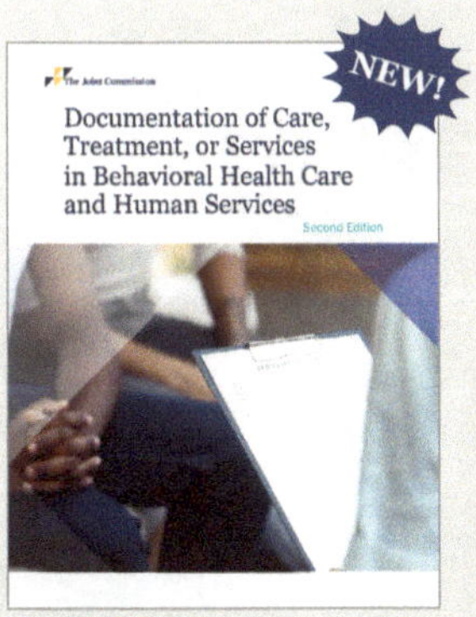

[Documentation of Care, Treatment, or Services in Behavioral Health Care, Second Edition]

BH23

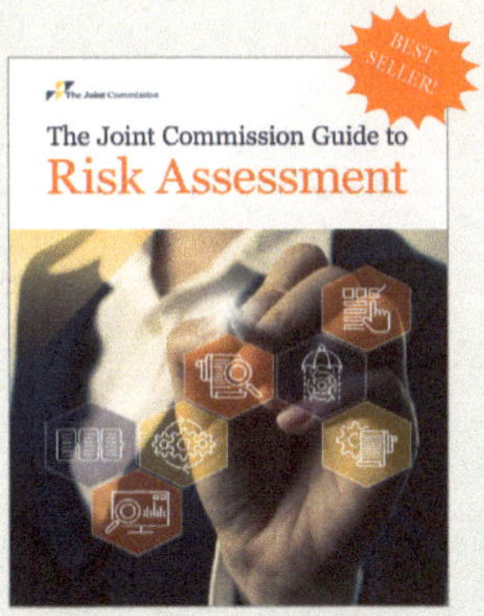

[The Joint Commission Guide to Risk Assessment]

JCRA21

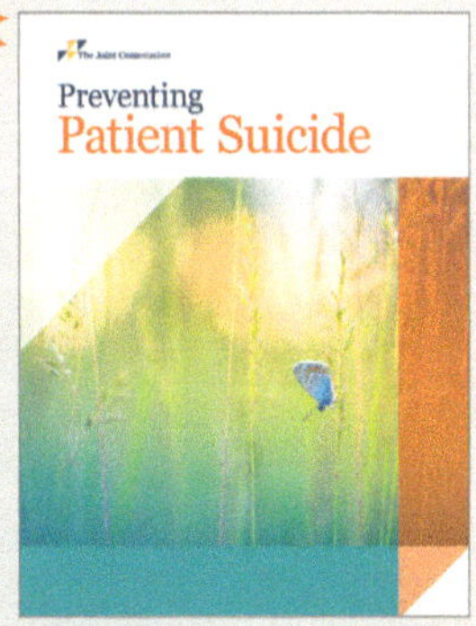

[Preventing Patient Suicide]

PPSU22

Performance Improvement and Patient Safety *continued*

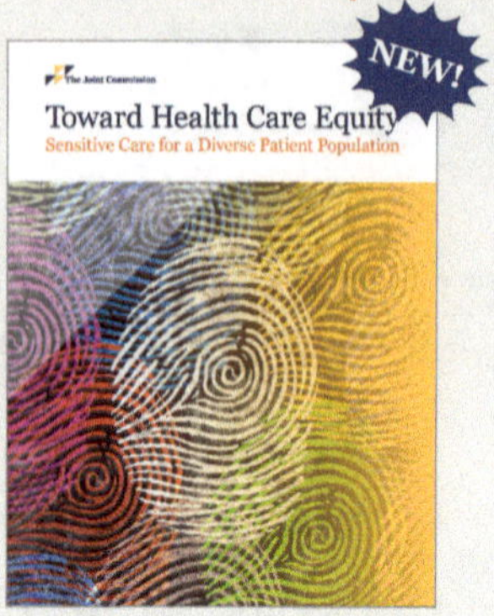

Toward Health Care Equity: Sensitive Care for a Diverse Patient Population
EBDCCH23SL

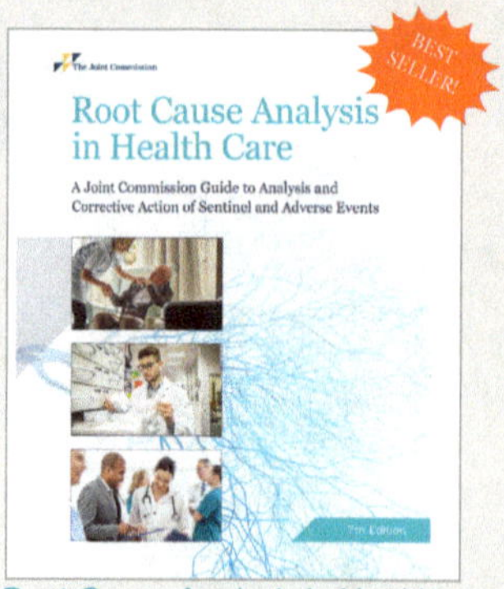

Root Cause Analysis in Health Care: A Joint Commission Guide to Analysis and Corrective Action of Sentinel and Adverse Events, Seventh Edition
RCA20

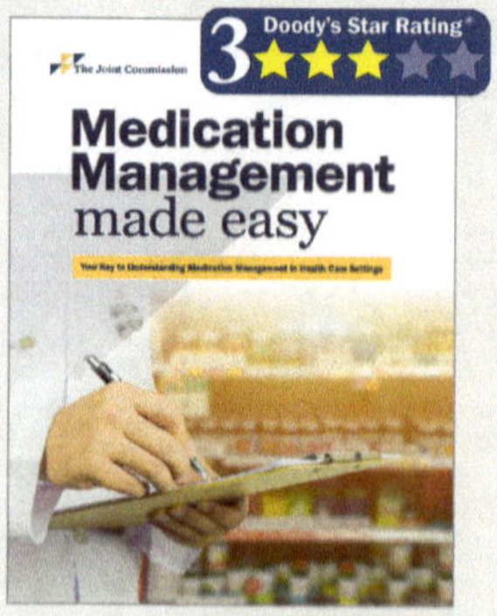

Medication Management Made Easy: Your Key to Understanding Medication Management in Health Care Settings
MMME21

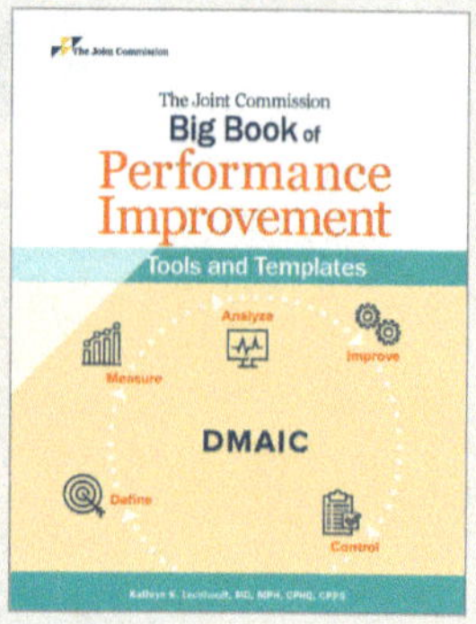

The Joint Commission Big Book of Performance Improvement Tools and Templates
JCPI19

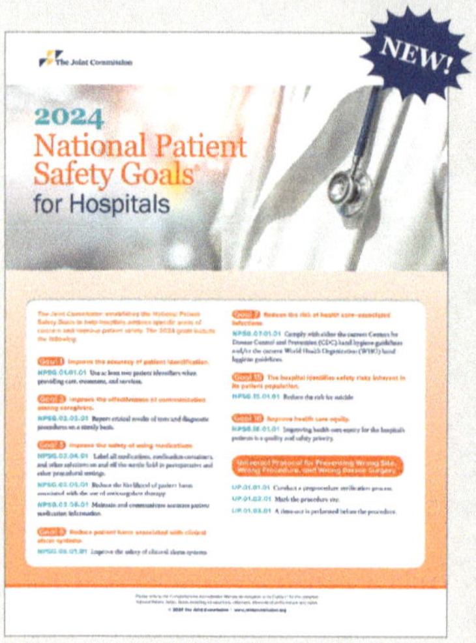

2024 National Patient Safety Goals® for Hospitals Products
Includes new health care equity goal!

Large 18"x24" Posters
NPSGH24

8.5"x11" Posters
NSPGHS24

Badge Buddies
SGBB24

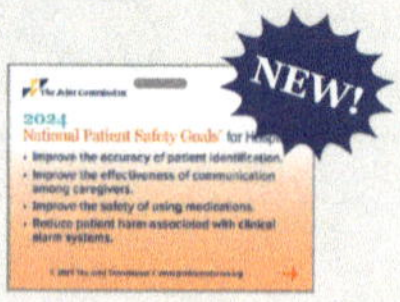

MORE TITLES

The Joint Commission Big Book of Tracer Questions
JCTQ17

The Joint Commission Big Book of MORE Tracer Questions
EBJCMTQ19

Strategies for Creating, Sustaining, and Improving a Culture of Safety in Health Care, Second Edition
SIHCS17

Front Line of Defense: The Role of Nurses in Preventing Sentinel Events, Third Edition
FLD18

Health Care Worker Safety Checklists: Protecting Those Who Serve
HCWS19

Digital Subscriptions

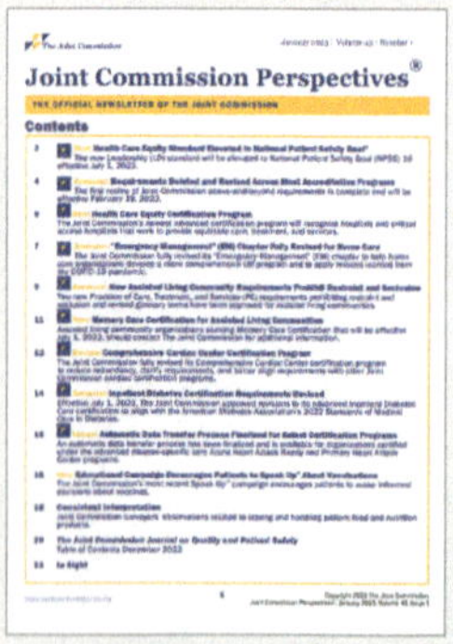

The Joint Commission Perspectives®
JCP1YOO
The official Joint Commission newsletter

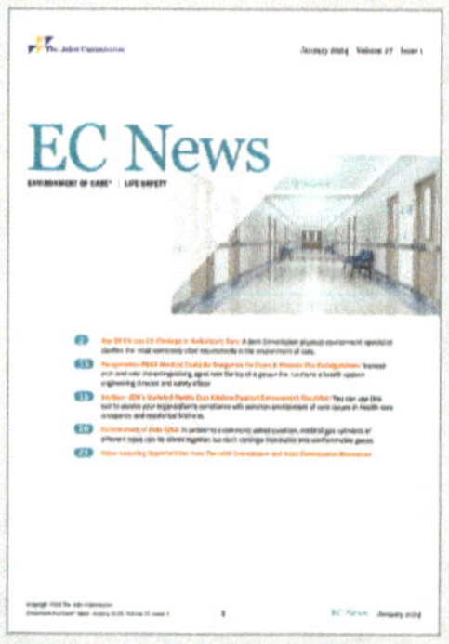

Environment of Care® News
ECN1YOO
Monthly newsletter for Environment of Care and Life Safety

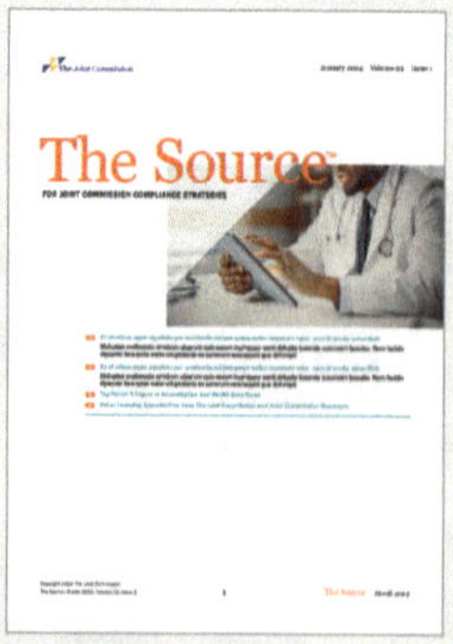

The Source™
TS1YOO
Monthly resource for Joint Commission compliance strategies

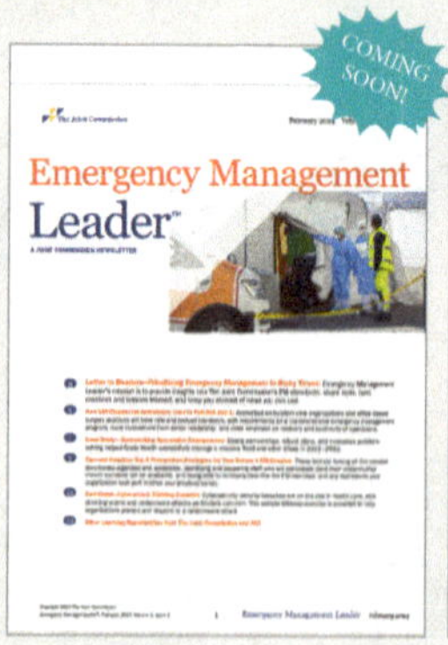

Emergency Management Leader™
EML1YOO
New bimonthly newsletter for EM compliance

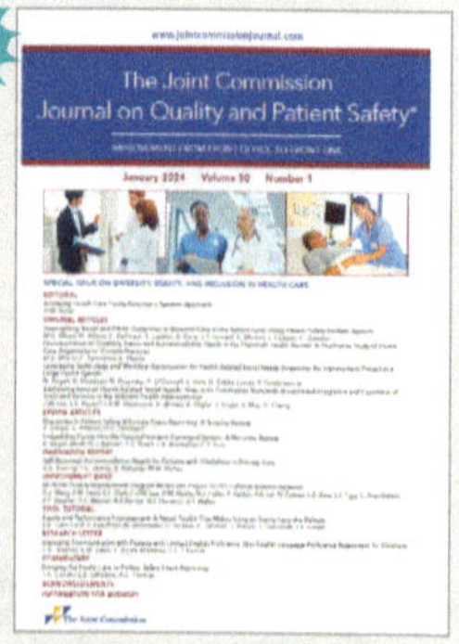

The Joint Commission Journal on Quality and Patient Safety®
Peer-reviewed articles featuring how-we-did-it success stories

Order online at www.jcrinc.com!

Additional Online Resources

Agency for Healthcare Research and Quality (AHRQ)
https://www.ahrq.gov/

American Chemical Society (ACS)
https://www.acs.org/

American College of Physicians (ACP)
https://www.acponline.org/

American Dental Association (ADA)
https://www.ada.org/

American Medical Association (AMA)
https://www.ama-assn.org/

American Nurses Association (ANA)
https://www.nursingworld.org/

American Society of Health-System Pharmacists (ASHP)
https://www.ashp.org/

ASPR [Administration for Strategic Preparedness and Response] Technical Resources, Assistance Center, and Information Exchange (TRACIE)
https://asprtracie.hhs.gov/

Association for the Advancement of Blood and Biotherapies (AABB)
https://www.aabb.org/

Association for the Advancement of Medical Instrumentation (AAMI)
https://www.aami.org/

Center for HICS [Hospital Incident Command System] Education & Training
https://www.calhospitalprepare.org/post/center-hics

Centers for Disease Control and Prevention (CDC)
https://www.cdc.gov/

> **National Healthcare Safety Network (NHSN)**
> https://www.cdc.gov/nhsn/index.html
>
> **National Institute for Occupational Safety and Health (NIOSH)**
> https://www.cdc.gov/niosh/index.htm

Centers for Medicare & Medicaid Services (CMS)
https://www.cms.gov/

> **State Operations Manual**
> https://www.cms.gov/regulations-and-guidance/guidance/manuals/downloads/som107ap_a_hospitals.pdf

Clinical and Laboratory Standards Institute (CLSI)
https://clsi.org/

Clinical Laboratory Improvement Amendments (CLIA)
https://www.cms.gov/medicare/quality/clinical-laboratory-improvement-amendments

Department of Health and Human Services (HHS)
https://www.hhs.gov/

Emergency Management Institute Independent Study Program
https://training.fema.gov/is/

Emergency Nurses Association
https://www.ena.org/

Federal Emergency Management Agency (FEMA)
https://www.fema.gov/

Institute for Healthcare Improvement (IHI)
https://www.ihi.org/

Institute for Safe Medication Practices (ISMP)
https://www.ismp.org/

The Joint Commission
https://www.jointcommission.org/

Antibiotic Stewardship Resources
https://www.jointcommission.org/resources/patient-safety-topics/infection-prevention-and-control/antibiotic-stewardship/

Fact Sheets
https://www.jointcommission.org/resources/news-and-multimedia/fact-sheets/#sort=%40itemtitle%20ascending

Interpreting Joint Commission Standards: FAQs
https://www.jointcommission.org/standards/standard-faqs/

Suicide Prevention Portal
https://www.jointcommission.org/resources/patient-safety-topics/suicide-prevention/

***Survey Activity Guide* (for accredited organizations, the *Survey Activity Guide* is available on the organization's *Joint Commission Connect®* extranet site)**

***Survey Activity Guide* for Ambulatory Care**
https://www.jointcommission.org/what-we-offer/accreditation/health-care-settings/ambulatory-health-care/prepare/snapshot-of-survey-day/

***Survey Activity Guide* for Assisted Living Community**
https://www.jointcommission.org/what-we-offer/accreditation/health-care-settings/assisted-living-community/prepare/snapshot-of-survey-day/

***Survey Activity Guide* for Behavioral Health Care and Human Services**
https://www.jointcommission.org/what-we-offer/accreditation/health-care-settings/behavioral-health-care/prepare/snapshot-of-survey-day/

***Survey Activity Guide* for Critical Access Hospital**
https://www.jointcommission.org/what-we-offer/accreditation/health-care-settings/critical-access-hospital/prepare/snapshot-of-survey-day/

***Survey Activity Guide* for Home Care**
https://www.jointcommission.org/what-we-offer/accreditation/health-care-settings/home-care/prepare/snapshot-of-survey-day/

***Survey Activity Guide* for Hospital**
https://www.jointcommission.org/what-we-offer/accreditation/health-care-settings/hospital/prepare/snapshot-of-survey-day/

***Survey Activity Guide* for Laboratory**
https://www.jointcommission.org/what-we-offer/accreditation/health-care-settings/laboratory-services/prepare/snapshot-of-survey-day/

***Survey Activity Guide* for Nursing Care Center**
https://www.jointcommission.org/what-we-offer/accreditation/health-care-settings/nursing-care-center/prepare/snapshot-of-survey-day/

National Center for Missing & Exploited Children
https://www.missingkids.org/home

National Fire Protection Association (NFPA)
https://www.nfpa.org/

National Institute on Aging
https://www.nia.nih.gov/

National Quality Measures Clearinghouse (NQMC)
https://psnet.ahrq.gov/issue/national-quality-measures-clearinghouse-nqmc

Occupational Safety and Health Administration (OSHA)
https://www.osha.gov/

Job Hazard Analysis
https://www.osha.gov/sites/default/files/publications/osha3071.pdf

Society of Gastroenterology Nurses and Associates (SGNA)
https://www.sgna.org/

Substance Abuse and Mental Health Services Administration (SAMHSA)
https://www.samhsa.gov/

US Department of Homeland Security (DHS)
https://www.dhs.gov/

US Department of Veterans Affairs (VA)
https://www.va.gov/

US Food and Drug Administration (FDA)
https://www.fda.gov/

Test Your Knowledge Answers

PART 1

Chapter 1

1. b, c, d
2. a
3. a
4. a, b
5. a
6. d
7. a
8. b

Chapter 2

1. a
2. a
3. b
4. a, b, c
5. b

PART 2

Chapter 3

1. b
2. a
3. d
4. c
5. c
6. a, b
7. c
8. b
9. c

Chapter 4

1. d
2. a
3. c
4. b

Chapter 5

1. c
2. b
3. b

4A. c
4B. b
5. b
6A. c
6B. a

Chapter 6

1. c
2. b
3. c
4. a, b, c, d
5. c

PART 3

Chapter 7

1A. Process
1B. Process
1C. Outcome
1D. Outcome
1E. Continuous variable
1F. Process
1G. Outcome
2. d
3. a, b

Chapter 8

1. b
2. c, d
3. c
4. a, b, c

PART 4

Chapter 9

1. b
2. a, b
3. a, b, c, d
4. a
5. d

Chapter 10

1. Activities to restore services are recovery; activities to build capacity are preparedness; activities to lessen impact are mitigation; activities implemented to react are response
2. c
3. c
4. c

Chapter 11

1. a
2. b
3. a, c
4. b
5. b, c

Chapter 12

1. Fire drills are fire safety; automatic sprinkler suppression system is life safety; fire-rated doors and doorway are life safety; RACE and PASS are fire safety
2. b
3. a, b

Chapter 13

1. a, b, c
2. b
3. a, b, c, d
4. b
5. b, c

Chapter 14

1. b, c, d
2. b, c
3. a
4. b

Chapter 15

1. b
2. b
3. a

Chapter 16

1. a, d
2. c
3. b
4. a
5. c
6. b
7. b, c
8. a
9. a

Chapter 17

1. a
2. b
3. c
4. b
5. a, b, c, d
6. c, d

Chapter 18

1. d
2. b
3. c
4. a, b, c, d
5. a, c
6. b
7. a

Chapter 19

1. b
2. c
3. a, b, c
4. c
5. b
6. c
7. a

Glossary

This glossary matches that in E-dition and the *Comprehensive Accreditation Manuals*

abuse
Intentional mistreatment that may cause either physical or psychological injury. *See also* neglect.

accountability measure
A measure that produces the greatest positive impact on care recipient outcomes when organizations improve on those outcomes. The measure meets these criteria:

- *Accuracy.* The measure accurately assesses whether the care process has actually been provided.
- *Adverse effects.* Implementing the measure has little or no chance of inducing unintended adverse effects.
- *Proximity.* The care process is closely connected to the outcome of the care recipient; there are few clinical processes that occur after the one that is measured and before the improved outcome occurs.
- *Research.* Strong scientific evidence demonstrates that performing the evidence-based care process improves health outcomes (either directly or by reducing risk of adverse outcomes).

Accreditation Participation Requirements (APR)
A standard that relates directly to the accreditation process and maintaining accreditation. APRs are included on E-dition® and in the hard-copy *Comprehensive Accreditation Manual*.

accreditation professional
A person responsible for helping to earn or maintain a health care organization's Joint Commission accreditation. This person may do any or all of the following: organize and oversee data collection, analysis, and reporting as outlined on E-dition and in the hard-copy *Comprehensive Accreditation Manual*; handle the accreditation application process; prepare for and act as liaison during the survey process; address any Requirements for Improvement (RFIs); and handle the Intracycle Monitoring (ICM) process.

action plan
A plan for addressing deficiencies that describes the planned action, when it will be implemented, and the associated measure(s) of effectiveness. *See also* Plan of Action (POA).

advance directive
A document or documentation allowing a person to give directions about future health care or to designate another person(s) to make health care decisions if

the individual loses decision-making capacity. Advance directives may include living wills, durable powers of attorney, do-not-resuscitate (DNR) orders, right-to-die documents, or similar documents listed in the Patient Self-Determination Act that express the person's preferences.

adverse drug event (ADE)
An injury resulting from a medical intervention related to a medication, including harm from an adverse drug reaction or a medication error. *See also* medication error.

adverse drug reaction (ADR)
A response to a medicinal product that is noxious and unintended and that occurs at doses normally used in humans for the prophylaxis, diagnosis, or treatment of disease or for the restoration, correction, or modification of physiological or psychological function.

adverse event
A patient safety event that resulted in harm to a care recipient.

assessment
An objective evaluation or appraisal of an individual's health , including acute and chronic conditions. The assessment gathers information through collection of data, observation, and physical examination. *See also* reassessment.

benchmarking
Continuous comparison of an organization's performance to that of tough competitors or industry leaders, or to similar activities in the organization, in order to find and implement ways to improve it.

best practices
Clinical, scientific, or professional practices that are recognized by a majority of professionals in a particular field as being exemplary. These practices are typically evidence based and consensus driven.

care planning (or planning for care)
Creating a plan of care that is individualized to a particular care recipient. The plan formulates strategies, goals, and objectives for care, treatment, or services. It may include narratives, policies and procedures, protocols, practice guidelines, clinical paths, care maps, or a combination of these.

care recipient/family education
A process of giving a care recipient and their family the knowledge or skills necessary for those individuals to take a more active role in managing the care recipient's health care needs.

chapter leader
A person assigned to assist the accreditation professional with a particular chapter of the *Comprehensive Accreditation Manual*. This person could be a departmental head or leader in a particular area, patient safety officer, nurse executive, director of performance improvement, chief of security, facility manager, and so on. The Joint Commission does not require the use of chapter leaders.

cleaning, disinfecting, and sterilizing
Methods used to prepare items for use in care, treatment, or services. *Cleaning* is the act of removing unwanted foreign matter or pollution. *Disinfecting* is a treatment to destroy or prevent the growth of harmful microorganisms. *Sterilizing* is the use of a physical or chemical procedure to destroy living microorganisms. *See also* reprocessing.

clinical care
The care, treatment, and services provided to a care recipient.

clinical leader
A clinician with essential knowledge in a clinical area who has responsibility in that area, including performance improvement.

clinical privileges
Authorization granted by the appropriate authority (for example, the governing body) to a physician or other licensed practitioner to provide specific care, treatment, or services in the organization within well-defined limits, based on the following factors: license, education, training, experience, competence, health status, and judgment.

close call
A patient safety event that did not reach a care recipient but posed a risk of harm; also called *near miss* or *good catch*.

comprehensive systematic analysis
A process for identifying basic or causal factors underlying variation in performance, including the occurrence or possible occurrence of a sentinel event. A root cause analysis is one type of comprehensive systematic analysis.

continuing care
Care, treatment, or services provided over time in various settings, programs, or services, from illness to wellness and spanning the illness-to-wellness continuum.

continuity of operations plan (COOP)
An uninterrupted ability of a health care organization to continue to provide essential or critical services and support, while maintaining organizational viability, before, during, and after an emergency or disaster incident.

contracted services
Services provided through a written agreement with another organization, agency, or person. The agreement specifies the services or personnel to be provided on behalf of the applicant organization and the fees to provide these services or personnel.

coordination of care
The process of coordinating care, treatment, or services provided by a health care organization, including referral to appropriate community resources and liaison with others (such as the individual's physician or other licensed practitioner, other health care organizations, or community services involved in care or services) to meet the ongoing identified needs of individuals, to ensure implementation of the plan of care, and to avoid unnecessary duplication of services.

corrective action plan

1. A detailed account of action taken by the organization to address specific areas of noncompliance submitted as part of the Evidence of Standards Compliance (ESC) submission following a Joint Commission survey.
2. The product of a root cause analysis that identifies the strategies that an organization intends to implement to reduce the risk of similar events occurring in the future. The plan addresses responsibility for implementation, oversight, pilot testing (as appropriate), time lines, and strategies for measuring the effectiveness of the actions.

credentialing

The process of obtaining, verifying, and assessing the qualifications of a physician or other licensed practitioner to provide care or services in or for a health care organization. *See also* designated equivalent source; primary source verification.

culture of safety

An environment in which safety is the top priority. In a culture of safety, not only are processes designed for optimal safety, but employees feel safe in reporting unsafe situations. Also referred to as a safety culture.

data

Raw facts and statistics collected together for reference or analysis. *See also* information; uniform data set.

deemed status, deeming authority

Status conferred by the Centers for Medicare & Medicaid Services (CMS) on an organization whose standards and survey process are determined by CMS to be equivalent to those of the Medicare program or other federal laws, such as the Clinical Laboratory Improvement Amendments of 1988 (CLIA '88). Accreditation is voluntary and seeking deemed status through accreditation is an option, not a requirement.

defend in place

A fire emergency strategy for health care occupancy in which occupants remain within the health care facility rather than being evacuated. This is accomplished by limiting the development and spread of a fire to the room of fire origin and reducing the need for occupant evacuation, except from the room of fire origin.

designated equivalent source

Selected agencies that have been determined to maintain a specific item(s) of credential(s) information that is identical to the information at the primary source. Some of the agencies may provide credential(s) information and services beyond what is identified below. Listing the names of these agencies does not constitute an endorsement. Designated equivalent sources include, but are not limited to, the following:

- The American Medical Association (AMA) Physician Masterfile for verification of a physician's United States and Puerto Rican medical school graduation and postgraduate education completion
- The American Board of Medical Specialties (ABMS) for verification of a physician's board certification

- The Educational Commission for Foreign Medical Graduates (ECFMG) for verification of a physician's graduation from a foreign medical school
- The American Osteopathic Association (AOA) Physician Database for pre-doctoral education accredited by the AOA Bureau of Professional Education; postdoctoral education approved by the AOA Council on Postdoctoral Training; postdoctoral education approved by the Accreditation Council for Graduate Medical Education (ACGME); and Osteopathic Specialty Board Certification
- The Federation of State Medical Boards (FSMB) for all actions against a physician's medical license
- The American Academy of Physician Assistants (AAPA) Profile for physician assistant education, provided through the AMA Physician Profile Service (https://profiles.ama-assn.org/amaprofiles/)
- National Commission on Certification of Physician Assistants (NCCPA) certification
- The National Board of Physicians and Surgeons (NBPAS) for verification of a physician's board certification.

See also credentialing.

discharge planning

A formalized process in a health care organization through which a program of continuing and follow-up care is planned and carried out for each care recipient.

documentation

1. Historical record of the care recipient's condition and encounters with the health care organization.
2. A required document or reference that goes beyond what's required to be in the record of care. Examples of documentation include written procedures, policies, written plans, bylaws, licenses, evidence of testing, data, performance improvement reports, medication labels, safety data sheets (SDSs), and meeting minutes.

drug diversion

The act of removing legal prescription drugs to an illegal channel of distribution or use.

Early Survey Policy

A policy that permits an organization to achieve accreditation in a two-survey process. The first survey is limited in scope, and successful completion results in Preliminary Accreditation. Organizations receiving Preliminary Accreditation under this policy are not recognized by the Centers for Medicare & Medicaid Services (CMS) to meet the requirements for Medicare certification. The second survey addresses all accreditation requirements, and successful completion results in full accreditation and recognition by CMS if requesting deemed status. The CMS Survey & Operations Group (SOG) location makes the final determination regarding an organization's Medicare participation and the effective date of participation.

E-dition®

A Web-based and fully searchable electronic manual that includes current Joint Commission accreditation standards, including all related content printed in the hard-copy *Comprehensive Accreditation Manual*, accessible through an organization's *Joint Commission Connect®* extranet site.

electronic health record (EHR)

A digital version of a care recipient's chart or record of care, which can be shared easily across various health care settings via computer networks. Also known as an *electronic medical record (EMR)*.

element of performance (EP)

Specific action(s), process(es), or structure(s) that must be implemented to achieve the goal of a standard. The scoring of EP compliance determines an organization's overall compliance with a standard.

emergency operations plan (EOP)

The organization's written document that describes the process it would implement for managing the consequences of emergencies, including natural and human-made disasters, that could disrupt the organization's ability to provide care, treatment, or services. Also known as *emergency management plan (EMP)*.

environmental tour

A routine comprehensive tour of the organization's facilities to evaluate environmental conditions and the effectiveness of current practice in managing environmental safety risks. This tour is not required by the standards.

environment of care

The physical environment of a health care organization, which includes the building itself and its grounds, utilities, medical equipment, and more. Some organizations refer to this as the EOC; The Joint Commission uses the acronym "EC."

epidemic

A disease, such as influenza, that spreads rapidly, attacks many people in a geographic area, causes a high rate of morbidity or mortality, and then subsides. *Epidemic* applies especially to infectious diseases, as in an epidemic of cholera, but is also applied to any disease, injury, or other health-related event, such as an epidemic of teenage suicide.

equivalency

A Joint Commission–approved alternate approach to a known *Life Safety Code®** deficiency that is mitigated by other building features so that the noncompliant condition is no longer identified as deficient. Equivalencies require submittal to and review by The Joint Commission. When The Joint Commission completes its analysis, the request is forwarded to the appropriate US Centers for Medicare & Medicaid Services (CMS) regional office for final disposition. The Joint Commission allows for two types of equivalencies:

---

* *Life Safety Code®* is a registered trademark of the National Fire Protection Association, Quincy, MA.

- Traditional equivalency, which requires field validation by a registered architect, a fire safety professional, or a fire marshal responsible for community fire safety.
- Fire Safety Evaluation System (FSES) equivalency, which is a formula-based approach that evaluates the entire building and deducts deficient conditions. If the net score is 0 or better, the building is considered "equalized."

evidence-based guidelines
Guidelines that have been scientifically developed based on recent literature review and are consensus-driven. Also known as *clinical practice guidelines*.

Evidence of Standards Compliance (ESC)
A report submitted by a surveyed organization, which details the action(s) that it took to bring itself into compliance with an accreditation requirement or clarifies why the organization believes that it was in compliance with the accreditation requirement for which it received a Requirement for Improvement. An ESC report must address compliance at the element of performance level. *See also* Requirement for Improvement (RFI).

executive committee
A committee made up of a few members of a board of directors. This committee is given authority to act quickly on issues that need to be addressed without having to wait for the next full board meeting. The committee can't be responsible for any of the board's major responsibilities; for example, the committee can't amend the bylaws or oversee an acquisition.

failure mode and effects analysis (FMEA)
An assessment that proactively examines a process in detail, including sequencing of events; assesses actual and potential risk, failure, or points of vulnerability; and, through a logical process, prioritizes areas for improvement based on the actual or potential impact (criticality) on care recipients.

fire rating
A classification indicating a material's resistance to fire, usually stated in terms of time before fire burns through the material.

fire safety
The minimum requirements for protecting against injury to life and/or property damage as a result of smoke, fire, and combustion, dependent on human intervention. Fire safety includes fire drills, means of egress, and clearly marked fire exits. *See also* life safety.

focused professional practice evaluation (FPPE)
The time-limited evaluation of physician or other licensed practitioner competence in performing a specific privilege. This process is implemented for all initially requested privileges and whenever a question arises regarding a practitioner's ability to provide safe, high-quality patient care. *See also* ongoing professional practice evaluation (OPPE).

Focused Standards Assessment (FSA)

A requirement of the accreditation process whereby an organization reviews its compliance with a selected subset of applicable Joint Commission accreditation requirements (including the applicable National Patient Safety Goals, a selection of standards that address accreditation program-specific high-risk areas, and the organization's Requirements for Improvement [RFIs] from its last triennial survey); completes and submits to The Joint Commission a Plan of Action (POA) for any accreditation requirement with which it is not in full compliance; and chooses whether to engage in a telephone discussion with a member of the Standards Interpretation Group staff to determine the acceptability of the POA or discuss any other area of concern. Alternatives for a full FSA submission include FSA Option 1 (attestation that an FSA was completed, but not submitted to The Joint Commission), Option 2 (onsite survey with documented findings), and Option 3 (on-site survey without documented findings). The FSA encourages organizations to be in continuous compliance with Joint Commission accreditation requirements and helps them to identify and manage risk. The organization retains the option to complete self-assessment with all applicable accreditation standards in the FSA tool, available on the organization's *Joint Commission Connect*® extranet site. *See also* Intracycle Monitoring (ICM). The FSA tool can also be used as a self-assessment tool by an organization preparing for its initial accreditation survey.

governing body

The group (usually a board of directors, or governance in a military hospital) that oversees the major business functions of an organization. Its responsibilities may include setting the budget, supervising the CEO and other senior leaders, and/or setting policies and goals for the organization.

hazardous medications

Drugs or substances that have the potential to cause harm on exposure. With prolonged exposure, these injuries can become critical and life threatening.

hazard vulnerability analysis (HVA)

A process for identifying potential emergencies and the direct and indirect effects these emergencies may have on the organization's operations and the demand for its services.

health care equity

When all people always experience safe, high-quality health care.

health care organization

An entity that provides medical or clinical care, treatment, and/or services. The Joint Commission surveys and accredits organizations in several health care settings: ambulatory care, assisted living communities, behavioral health care and human services, critical access hospitals, home care, hospitals, laboratories, nursing care centers, and office-based surgery practices.

health literacy

The degree to which individuals have the capacity to obtain, process, and understand basic health information and services needed to make appropriate health decisions.

health-related social needs

Care recipients need to (1) have a place to live, (2) be able to afford their medications, (3) be able to afford food to avoid adverse drug reactions, and (4) have transportation to get to appointments.

high-alert medications

Medications that bear a heightened risk of causing significant harm to care recipients when they are used in error.

history and physical (H&P)

Information gathered about an individual using a holistic approach for the purpose of establishing a diagnosis and developing a plan for care, treatment, or services to address physical health issues. The history may include information about previous illnesses; previous medical or surgical interventions and response to treatment; family health history; and social, cultural, economic, and lifestyle issues that may affect the individual's health and well-being. The physical involves the physical examination of the individual's body by the following means: inspection, palpation, percussion, and auscultation. When used in concert with behavioral health care and human services, the history and physical may be used to rule out physical causes for behavioral health conditions or to assess the impact of a medical diagnosis or treatment on a behavioral health condition or current situation.

Immediate Threat to Health or Safety

A threat that represents immediate risk and has or may potentially have serious adverse effects on the health or safety of the patient, resident, or individual served. These threats are identified by the surveyor.

infection control risk assessment (ICRA)

A multidisciplinary, organizational, documented process that provides information about risk mitigation related to construction projects including but not limited to air quality, water quality, utility system function, traffic flow, waste disposal, and other issues.

infectious/medical waste

Waste materials generated at health care facilities, including a broad range of materials, from used needles and soiled dressings to medical devices and radioactive materials.

information

Data that have been processed, interpreted, and given context so they can be useful. *See also* data.

informed consent

Agreement or permission accompanied by full notice about the care, treatment, or service that is the subject of the consent. A patient must be apprised of the nature, risks, and alternatives of a medical procedure or treatment before the physician or other licensed practitioner begins any such course. After receiving this information, the patient then either consents to or refuses such a procedure or treatment.

interdisciplinary team

A group of individuals from different disciplines or professions who collaborate to plan, treat, or provide care or services to an individual.

Intracycle Monitoring (ICM)

A process to help accredited organizations at various touch points in the triennial accreditation cycle with their continuous compliance efforts. The process involves access to an ICM Profile available on the organization's *Joint Commission Connect*® extranet site. The ICM Profile identifies high-risk areas and related standards areas and displays them within a Focused Standards Assessment (FSA) tool, which allows organizations to conduct a self-assessment of standards to identify and manage risk in the organization. *See also* Focused Standards Assessment (FSA).

licensed practitioner

An individual who is licensed and qualified to direct or provide care, treatment, and services in accordance with state law and regulation, applicable federal law and regulation, and organizational policy.

life safety

The minimum requirements for protecting against injury to life and/or property damage as a result of smoke, fire, and combustion, dependent on building features. Life safety includes smoke alarm and sprinkler systems, construction, hardware, and layout (design elements). *See also* fire safety.

Life Safety Code®

A set of standards for the construction and operation of buildings intended to provide a reasonable degree of safety during fires. These standards are prepared, published, and periodically revised by the National Fire Protection Association and adopted by The Joint Commission to evaluate health care organizations under its life safety management program. *See also* occupancy.

means of egress

A continuous and unobstructed way of travel from any point in a building or other structure to a public way consisting of three separate and distinct parts: the exit access, the exit, and the exit discharge.

medical equipment, devices, and supplies

Elements used to deliver clinical care, treatment, or services. Medical equipment is fixed or portable equipment used in the care continuum. Medical devices include any instrument, apparatus, implant, in vitro reagent, or similar or related article that is used to diagnose, prevent, or treat disease or other conditions. Medical supplies are items that are typically disposable, such as bandages, sterile drapes, and suture materials. As such, they differ from permanent or durable items, such as medical equipment and devices.

medical record

See record of care.

medical staff

The group of physicians and other licensed practitioners privileged through the organized medical staff process that is subject to the medical staff bylaws. This group may include others, such as retired practitioners who no longer practice in the organization but who wish to continue their membership in the group, courtesy staff, scientific staff, and so forth. Not to be confused with the organized medical staff.

medical staff bylaws
A document or group of documents adopted by the voting members of the organized medical staff and approved by the governing body that defines the rights, responsibilities, and accountabilities of the medical staff and various officers, persons, and groups within the structure of the organized medical staff; the self-governance functions of the organized medical staff; and the working relationship with and accountability to the governing body of the organized medical staff.

medication error
A preventable event that may cause or lead to inappropriate medication use or harm to a care recipient while the medication is in the control of the health care professional, care recipient, or consumer. Such events may be related to professional practice, health care products, procedures, and systems, including prescribing; order communication; product labeling, packaging, and nomenclature; compounding; dispensing; distribution; administration; education; monitoring; and use. *See also* adverse drug event (ADE).

medication reconciliation
The process of identifying the medications currently taken by an individual. These medications are compared to newly ordered medications, and discrepancies are identified and resolved.

National Patient Safety Goals® (NPSG)
Standards requiring specific actions that an accredited organization is required to take to prevent medical errors. NPSGs comprise simple, proven steps determined by a panel of national safety experts to reduce the frequency of significant medical errors.

near miss
See close call.

neglect
The absence of the minimal services or resources required to meet basic needs. Neglect includes withholding or inadequately providing medical care and, consistent with usual care, treatment, or services, food and hydration (without approval from the individual, physician or other licensed practitioner, or surrogate), clothing, or good hygiene. It may also include placing an individual in unsafe or unsupervised conditions. *See also* abuse.

nurse executive
A registered professional nurse who is responsible for the full-time, direct supervision of nursing services and who is currently licensed by the state in which they practice. Attributes of this position may be further defined in regulatory statutes.

occupancy

The purpose for which a building or portion thereof is used or intended to be used. Depending on the organization, occupancies may include ambulatory health care occupancy, business occupancy, health care occupancy, and residential occupancy.

- **ambulatory health care occupancy** An occupancy used to provide services or treatment to four or more patients (or one or more patients in an ambulatory surgical center that elects to use The Joint Commission deemed status option) at the same time that either (1) renders them incapable of providing their own means of self-preservation in an emergency or (2) provides outpatient surgical treatment requiring general anesthesia.
- **business occupancy** An occupancy used to provide outpatient care, treatment, day treatment, or other services that does not meet the criteria in the ambulatory health care occupancy definition (for example, three or fewer individuals at the same time who are either rendered incapable of self-preservation in an emergency or are undergoing general anesthesia). For ambulatory surgical centers that elect to use The Joint Commission deemed status option, treatment of one or more incapacitated patients renders the area an ambulatory health care occupancy.
- **health care occupancy** An occupancy used for purposes such as medical or other treatment or care of persons suffering from physical or mental illness, disease, or infirmity; and for the care of infants, convalescents, or infirm aged persons. Health care occupancies provide sleeping facilities for four or more occupants and are occupied by persons who are mostly incapable of self-preservation because of age, physical or mental disability, or security measures not under the occupant's control. Health care occupancies include hospitals, critical access hospitals, skilled nursing homes, and limited care facilities. *See also* Life Safety Code.

occupational exposure

Exposure to potentially harmful chemical, physical, or biological agents within the workplace or as a result of performing job duties.

ongoing professional practice evaluation (OPPE)

A document summary of ongoing data collected for the purpose of assessing a physician's or other licensed practitioner's clinical competence and professional behavior. The information gathered during this process is factored into decisions to maintain, revise, or revoke existing privilege(s) prior to or at the end of the two-year license and privilege renewal cycle. *See also* focused professional practice evaluation (FPPE).

organized medical staff

The self-governing body of the medical staff. It operates under the medical staff bylaws, which are approved by the governing body. The members of the organized medical staff are licensed to make independent diagnosis and treatment decisions.

outcome measure

A tool used to assess data that indicates the results of performance or nonperformance of a function or procedure.

patient safety event

An event, incident, or condition that could have resulted or did result in harm to a care recipient.

performance improvement (PI)

The systematic process of detecting and analyzing performance problems, designing and developing interventions to address the problems, implementing the interventions, evaluating the results, and sustaining improvement.

performance measure

A quantitative tool (for example, rate, ratio, index, percentage) that provides an indication of an organization's performance in relation to a specified process or outcome.

personal protective equipment (PPE)

Equipment worn to minimize exposure to serious workplace injuries and illnesses that may result from contact with chemical, radiological, infectious, toxic, physical, or other workplace hazards. PPE may include gloves, eye protection, face masks, respirators, isolation gowns, and full body suits.

Plan for Improvement (PFI)

For purposes of Joint Commission accreditation, an organization's written statement that details the procedures to be taken and time frames to correct existing *Life Safety Code*® deficiencies, as identified in the Life Safety Assessment portion of the Joint Commission survey. The PFI is specific to life safety within the environment of care and shouldn't be confused with a Plan of Action (POA). *See also* Survey-Related Plan for Improvement (SPFI).

Plan of Action (POA)

A plan detailing the action(s) that an organization will take to come into compliance with a Joint Commission accreditation requirement. A POA must be completed for each element of performance associated with a non-compliant accreditation requirement. *See also* action plan; Plan for Improvement (PFI).

plan of care

See care planning.

point-of-care testing (POCT)

Analytical testing performed at sites outside the traditional laboratory environment, usually at or near where care is delivered to individuals. Testing may be categorized as waived, moderate, or high complexity under the Clinical Laboratory Improvement Amendments of 1988 (CLIA '88). Testing may range from simple waived procedures, such as fecal occult blood, to more sophisticated chemical analyzers. Guided by CLIA requirements, this testing may be under the control of the main laboratory, another specialized laboratory (for example, for arterial blood gas), or the nursing service (for example, for glucose meters). Point-of-care testing may also be known as alternative site testing, decentralized laboratory testing, or distributed site testing.

primary source verification

Verification of a physician's or other licensed practitioner's reported qualifications by the original source or an approved agent of that source. Methods for conducting primary source verification of credentials include direct correspondence, documented telephone verification, secure electronic verification from the original qualification source, or reports from credentials verification organizations (CVOs) that meet Joint Commission requirements. *See also* credentialing.

privileging

The process whereby the specific scope and content of patient care services (that is, clinical privileges) are authorized for a physician or other licensed practitioner by a health care organization based on evaluation of the individual's credentials and performance.

process measure

A measure focused on a process that leads to a particular outcome, meaning that a scientific basis exists for believing that the process, when executed well, will increase the probability of achieving a desired outcome.

protected health information (PHI)

Information about the health status, treatment, and any health care payments that can be linked to a specific individual.

reassessment

Ongoing data collection, which begins on initial assessment, comparing the most recent data with the data collected at earlier assessments. *See also* assessment.

record of care

1. An account compiled by physicians and other health care professionals of a variety of health information, such as assessment findings, treatment details, and progress notes.
2. Data obtained from the records or documentation maintained on a patient or resident in any health care setting (for example, hospital, home care, nursing care center, licensed practitioner office). The record includes automated and paper medical record systems.

reprocessing

A detailed, multistep approach for the cleaning, disinfecting, and sterilizing of reusable medical devices so they can be safely used on more than one care recipient. *See also* cleaning, disinfecting, and sterilizing.

Requirement for Improvement (RFI)

A recommendation that is required to be addressed in an organization's Evidence of Standards Compliance for the organization to retain its accreditation. Failure to adequately address an RFI after two opportunities may result in a recommendation to place the organization in Accreditation with Follow-up Survey. *See also* Evidence of Standards Compliance (ESC).

restraint

1. Any method (chemical or physical) of restricting an individual's freedom of movement, including seclusion, physical activity, or normal access to their body that (1) is not a usual and customary part of a medical diagnostic or treatment procedure to which the individual or their legal representative has consented, (2) is not indicated to treat the individual's medical condition or symptoms, or (3) does not promote the individual's independent functioning.
2. For hospitals and rehabilitation and psychiatric distinct part units in critical access hospitals that elect The Joint Commission deemed status option: 42 CFR 482.13(e)(1) Any manual method, physical or mechanical device, material, or equipment that immobilizes or reduces the ability of a patient to move his or her arms, legs, body, or head freely; or 42 CFR 482.13(e)(1)(i)(B) (A restraint is—) A drug or medication when it is used as a restriction to manage the patient's behavior or restrict the patient's freedom of movement and is not a standard treatment or dosage for the patient's condition. 42 CFR 482.13(e)(1)(i)(c) A restraint does not include devices, such as orthopedically prescribed devices, surgical dressings or bandages, protective helmets, or other methods that involve the physical holding of a patient for the purpose of conducting routine physical examinations or tests, or to protect the patient from falling out of bed, or to permit the patient to participate in activities without the risk of physical harm (this does not include a physical escort).

risk assessment, proactive

An assessment that examines a process in detail including sequencing of events, actual and potential risks, and failure or points of vulnerability and that prioritizes, through a logical process, areas for improvement based on the actual or potential impact (that is, criticality) of care, treatment, or services provided.

root cause analysis (RCA)

See comprehensive systematic analysis.

safety data sheet (SDS)

A sheet provided by the manufacturer that includes details about a substance's hazards. Employers must make sure that SDSs are readily accessible to employees. Formerly known as a *material safety data sheet*.

seclusion

1. The involuntary confinement of an individual in a room alone, for any period of time, from which the individual is physically prevented from leaving. Seclusion does not include involuntary confinement for legally mandated but nonclinical purposes, such as the confinement of a person who is facing serious criminal charges or who is serving a criminal sentence.
2. For hospitals and rehabilitation and psychiatric distinct part units in critical access hospitals that elect The Joint Commission deemed status option: The involuntary confinement of a patient alone in a room or area from which the patient is physically prevented from leaving. Seclusion may be used only for the management of violent or self-destructive behavior. (42 CFR 48 2.13(e)(1)(ii))

sentinel event

A patient safety event (not primarily related to the natural course of the patient's illness or underlying condition) that reaches a patient and results in death, severe harm (regardless of duration of harm), or permanent harm (regardless of severity of harm). Sentinel events are a subcategory of adverse events.

smoke compartment

A space within a building enclosed by smoke barriers on all sides, including the top and bottom.

staff

All people who provide care, treatment, or services in the organization, including licensed practitioners; permanent, temporary, part-time personnel; contract employees; volunteers; and health profession students.

standard

A principle of patient safety and quality of care that a well-run organization meets. A standard defines the performance expectations, structures, or processes that must be substantially in place in an organization to enhance the quality of care, treatment, or services.

standard precautions

Preventive and control measures to protect against potential exposure to infectious diseases.

surveillance

Systematic method of collecting, consolidating, and analyzing data concerning the frequency or pattern of, and causes or factors associated with, a given disease, injury, or other health condition. Data analysis is followed by the dissemination of that information to those who can improve outcomes. Examples of surveillance data can include ventilator associated pneumonia, antibiotic prophylaxis, hemodialysis catheter infections, implant infections, surgical site infections, hand hygiene, drug resistant organisms (MRSA, VRE), equipment sterile processing, vaccinations, urinary tract infections, and health care worker immunization.

Survey Analysis for Evaluating Risk® (*SAFER*®) Matrix

A tool that gives a visual representation of the risk level of each Requirement for Improvement (RFI). Each observation reported by a surveyor is plotted on the *SAFER* Matrix according to the risk level of the finding. The risk level is determined according to two factors: (1) the likelihood of the finding to cause harm to patients, staff, and/or visitors, and (2) the scope at which the finding was observed.

Survey-Related Plan for Improvement (SPFI)

An organization's written plan to resolve, within 60 days, an organization's deficiency with aspects of the *Life Safety Code*®, as identified in the Life Safety Assessment portion of the on-site Joint Commission survey. *See also* Plan for Improvement (PFI).

time-out
An immediate pause by the entire surgical team to confirm the correct patient, procedure, and site before performing an invasive procedure. *See also* Universal Protocol.

tissue adverse events
Injuries sustained by a care recipient due to a negative reaction to introduction of a foreign tissue, including disease transmission and infection.

tracer
A process used by surveyors to analyze an organization's systems by following or "tracing" an individual through the care, treatment, and services process.

transition of care
When an individual is moved from one health care setting to another.

transmission-based precautions
Infection prevention and control measures to protect against exposure to a suspected or identified pathogen. These precautions are specific and based on the way the pathogen is transmitted. Categories include contact, droplet, airborne, and a combination of these.

uniform data set
A collection of related information based on accepted terms and definitions. *See also* data.

Universal Protocol
A procedure to prevent wrong site, wrong procedure, and wrong person surgery through preprocedure verification, site marking, and a time-out. It's applicable to all invasive procedures, surgical and nonsurgical. Universal Protocol (UP) standards are included in the "National Patient Safety Goals" (NPSG) chapter of the *Comprehensive Accreditation Manual*. *See also* time-out.

waived testing
Tests that meet the Clinical Laboratory Improvement Amendments of 1988 (CLIA '88) requirements for waived tests and are cleared by the Food and Drug Administration for home use. These tests employ methodologies that are so simple and accurate that the likelihood of erroneous results is negligible, or they pose no risk of harm to the patient, resident, or individual served if the test is performed incorrectly.

workplace violence
An act or threat occurring at the workplace that can include any of the following: verbal, nonverbal, written, or physical aggression; threatening, intimidating, harassing, or humiliating words or actions; bullying; sabotage; sexual harassment; physical assaults; or other behaviors of concern involving staff, licensed practitioners, patients, or visitors.

Index

A

B

C

D

E

F

G

H

I

J

L

M

N

O

P

Q

R

S

T

U

V